THE CHINESE MEDICINE
COMPANION

Inspiring | Educating | Creating | Entertaining

First Published in 2020 by Fair Winds Press, an imprint of The Quarto Group, 100 Cummings Center, Suite 265-D, Beverly, MA 01915, USA.
T (978) 282-9590 F (978) 283-2742 QuartoKnows.com

Fair Winds Press titles are also available at discount for retail, wholesale, promotional, and bulk purchase. For details, contact the Special Sales Manager by email at specialsales@quarto.com or by mail at The Quarto Group, Attn: Special Sales Manager, 100 Cummings Center, Suite 265-D, Beverly, MA 01915, USA.

24 23 22 21 20 1 2 3 4 5

ISBN: 978-1-59233-989-1

Digital edition published in 2020
eISBN: 978-1-63159-977-4

The information in this book previously appeared in *The New Chinese Medicine Handbook* by Misha Ruth Cohen (Fair Winds Press, 2015).

Library of Congress Cataloging-in-Publication Data under *The New Chinese Medicine Handbook*.

Design: Merideth Harte
Page Layout: Merideth Harte
Illustration: William Michael Wanke and Shutterstock

Printed in China

THE
CHINESE
MEDICINE
COMPANION

A MODERN GUIDE TO ANCIENT HEALING

MISHA RUTH COHEN, O.M.D., L.AC.

CONTENTS

PREFACE

What is new in Integrated Chinese Medicine?

At first glance, there is nothing new. Chinese medicine has developed continuously over thousands of years. Chinese medicine philosophy states that everything constantly changes. Yin becomes Yang, and Yang becomes Yin. However, Integrated Chinese Medicine takes this concept of constant change and distinguishes it by incorporating modern medicine within the ancient philosophy of Chinese medicine.

First, Integrated Chinese Medicine is a partnership between ancient Chinese medicine wisdom and the insight of Western medicine. Second, with expanded access to all kinds of research and information due to the Internet, apps, and other modern technological advances, there is much more readily available knowledge. Within this overabundance of information, there is good and bad, true and false, and at times, it is hard to tell the difference. With Integrated Chinese Medicine, I can help you make sense of this morass of information and help you choose what actually works and what is safe. Third, you are in charge of your own healing process. Integrated Chinese Medicine, as shown in this book, gives you tools to make your own decisions and become supported as the captain of your healing team, with practitioners as your facilitators and catalysts.

You don't need to see a Chinese medicine practitioner or come to our clinic to reap the benefits of Integrated Chinese Medicine. You can use many self-care techniques to help you get started along your path to wholeness *today*.

Self-care practices can make a dramatic and immediate difference in the quality of your life even before you have explored the Chinese medicine concepts on which Integrated Chinese Medicine is based. Self-care therapies are *not* second best. I believe that they should be 80 percent of all care. They're the most important part of any journey toward wholeness. You can't arrive there unless you bring yourself along.

CHAPTER 1

THE PHYSIOLOGY AND ANATOMY OF CHINESE MEDICINE

C hinese medicine is a system of preserving health and curing disease that treats the mind/body/spirit as a whole. Its goal is to maintain or restore harmony and balance in all parts of the human being and also between the human being and the environment.

Each of Chinese medicine's healing arts—from dietary therapy to acupuncture—is designed to be integrated into daily life. Together, they offer the opportunity to live in harmony and to maintain wholeness. In fact, for all of Chinese medicine's power to heal the body, its focus is on preventive care. In ancient China, doctors were paid only when their patients were healthy. When patients became ill, obviously the doctors hadn't done their job.

The Role of the Tao

Chinese medicine's focus on maintaining wholeness and harmony of the mind/body/spirit emerges from the philosophy of the Tao, which is sometimes translated as "the infinite origin" or the "unnameable."

The guiding principles of the Tao are:

- Everything in the universe is part of the whole.

- Everything has its opposite.

- Everything is evolving into its opposite.

- The extremes of one condition are equal to its opposite.

- All antagonisms are complementary.

- There is no beginning and no end, yet whatever has a beginning has an end.

- Everything changes; nothing is absolute.

This dynamic balance between opposing forces, known as Yin/Yang, is the ongoing process of creation and destruction. It is the natural order of the universe and of each person's inner being.

To Westerners, Yin/Yang is most easily understood as a symbol for equilibrium, but in Chinese philosophy and medicine, it is not symbolic. It is as concrete as flesh and blood. It exists as an entity, a force, a quality, and a characteristic. It lives within the body, in the life force (Qi), in each Organ System.

The Forms of Qi

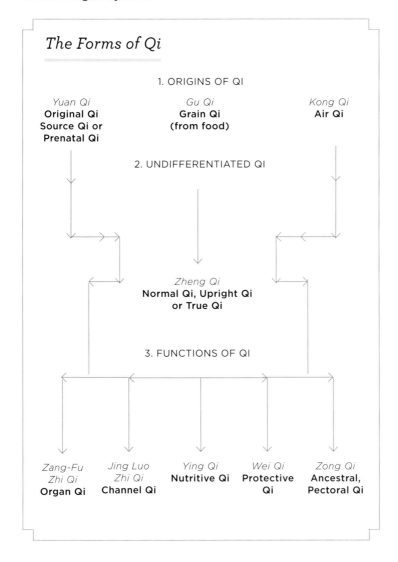

1. ORIGINS OF QI

Yuan Qi
Original Qi
Source Qi or
Prenatal Qi

Gu Qi
Grain Qi
(from food)

Kong Qi
Air Qi

2. UNDIFFERENTIATED QI

Zheng Qi
Normal Qi, Upright Qi
or True Qi

3. FUNCTIONS OF QI

Zang-Fu
Zhi Qi
Organ Qi

Jing Luo
Zhi Qi
Channel Qi

Ying Qi
Nutritive Qi

Wei Qi
Protective
Qi

Zong Qi
Ancestral,
Pectoral Qi

When the dynamic balance of Yin/Yang is disturbed, disharmony afflicts the mind/body/spirit, and disease can take root. Each symptom of Yin/Yang disharmony tells the trained practitioner about what's going on in the inner workings of a person's body. Once a disharmony is identified, the Chinese medicine practitioner addresses the entire web of interconnected responses in mind/body/spirit that are triggered by the presence of disharmony. Healing is achieved by rebalancing Yin and Yang and restoring harmony in the whole person.

Chinese medicine conceives of wellness and disease differently than Western medicine does, and it also describes the internal workings of the body in ways you may not be used to. In place of individual organs, blood vessels, and nerves, Chinese medicine identifies the body's Essential Substances, Organ Systems, and Channels.

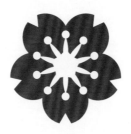

Essential Substances

The Essential Substances, which have an impact on and are impacted by both the Organ Systems and the Channels, are called Qi, Shen, Jing, Xue, and Jin-Ye.

QI

Qi (*chee*) is the basic life force that pulses through everything in the universe. Organic and inorganic matter are composed of and defined by Qi. Within each person, Qi warms the body, retains the body's fluids and organs, fuels the transformation of food into other substances such as Xue, protects the body from disease, and empowers movement.

We use the Chinese word for this substance because there is no precise English translation for the word or the concepts it contains. If you want to think of Qi as the energy that creates and animates material and spiritual being, you will come close to understanding Qi. As you delve more deeply into Chinese medicine, you will begin to identify how Qi lives within you and fuels your very existence. You'll find Qi is most accurately defined by its function and its impact.

Where does Qi come from and where does it go? We are all born with Qi. We can preserve, create, or deplete it by the air we breathe, the food we eat, and the way in which we live within our mind/body/spirit. There are many forms of Qi, which all work together.

SHEN

Shen (*shen*) is consciousness, thoughts, emotions, and senses, which make us uniquely human. Its harmonious flow is essential to good health. Originally transmitted into a fetus from both parents, Shen must be continuously nourished after birth.

JING

Jing (*jing*) is often translated as *essence*, the fluid that nurtures growth and development. We are born with Prenatal or Congenital Jing, inherited from our parents. Jing defines our basic constitution, along with Original Qi. Acquired Jing is transformed from food by the Stomach and Spleen, and it constantly replenishes the Prenatal Jing, which is consumed as we age.

Prenatal Jing gives rise to Qi, but during our lifetime, as Jing changes, it is dependent on Qi. Qi is Yang; Jing is Yin. Qi and Jing are joined in the process of aliveness. While Qi is the energy associated with any movement, Jing is the substance associated with the slow movement of organic change.

Prenatal Jing is our genetic capability, but whether we reach our genetic capability depends on how much Qi we are able to nurture. Think of a child whose parents are 6 feet (1.8 m) tall. If that child is malnourished, he or she will never reach the height conveyed by genetic potential. But if there is an ample supply of food, the child can grow fully. In the same way, if there is enough Qi, the possibilities of Jing can become realized.

XUE

The Chinese word Xue (*sch-whey*) is a much more precise description of this bodily substance than blood, which is the common English translation. Xue is not confined to the blood vessels, nor does it contain only plasma and red and white blood cells. Xue carries the Shen. Xue also moves along the Channels in the body where Qi flows.

Xue is produced by food that is collected and mulched in the Stomach, refined by the Spleen into a purified Essence (Acquired Jing), and then transported upward to the Lung,

The Production of Xue

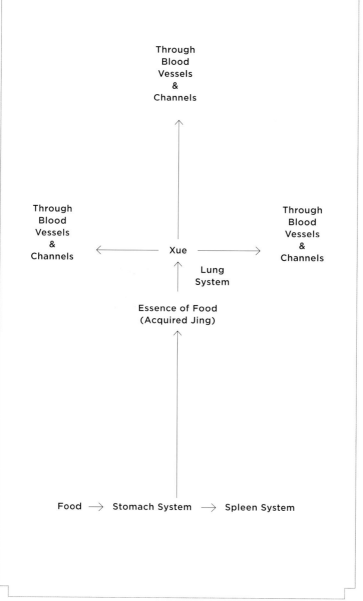

Through
Blood
Vessels
&
Channels

Through
Blood
Vessels
&
Channels

Xue

Through
Blood
Vessels
&
Channels

Lung
System

Essence of Food
(Acquired Jing)

Food ⟶ Stomach System ⟶ Spleen System

where Nutritive Qi begins to turn Jing into Xue. At the Lung, Jing combines with air and produces Xue. Qi propels Xue through the body.

Xue is intertwined with many body functions:

- Xue depends on the Heart System for its harmonious, smooth circulation.

- The Liver System stores Xue.

- The Spleen System governs Xue. The retentive properties of Spleen Qi keep Xue within its designated pathways.

- Qi creates and moves Xue and holds it in place. The Chinese saying is, "Qi is the commander of Xue."

- Xue in turn nourishes the Organ Systems that produce and regulate the Qi. It is also said that Xue is the mother of Qi.

JIN-YE

Jin-Ye (*jin-yee*), the Chinese word for all fluids other than Xue, includes sweat, urine, mucus, saliva, and other secretions such as bile and gastric acid. Jin-Ye is produced by digestion of food. Organ Qi regulates it. Certain forms of what is called Refined Jin-Ye help produce Xue.

These Five Essential Substances are the primordial soup from which life emerges and in which harmony and disharmony coexist. In Chinese medicine, reading the condition of these substances is an important part of diagnosis and treatment.

The Organ Systems

Chinese medicine talks about Organ Systems—not the individual, anatomical organs that are identified by Western medicine. Each Organ System governs specific body tissues, emotional states, and activities, and each Organ System is associated with and influenced by the Essential Substances and Channels.

- Every Organ System is governed by Organ Qi and influences the balance of Qi. This energy creates the Organ Systems' impact on the mind/body/spirit.

- The Essential Substances—Qi, Shen, Jing, Xue, and Jin-Ye—infuse each Organ System with energy and shape its characteristics.

- Some Organ Systems are Yin, and other Organ Systems are Yang. Together, they are called the Zang-Fu Organs, and they form a harmonious balance that sustains life.

ZANG (YIN) AND FU (YANG) ORGAN SYSTEMS

Zang (Yin)	Fu (Yang)
Kidney	Gallbladder
Spleen	Stomach
Liver	Small Intestine
Lung	Large Intestine
Heart	Urinary Bladder
Pericardium	Triple Burner

In general, Zang Organs are associated with pure substances—Qi, Xue, Jing, Shen, and Jin-Ye. Fu Organ Systems govern the digestion of food and the elimination of waste. But the division between Zang (Yin) and Fu (Yang) organs is not black and white. Each organ, whether Zang (Yin) or Fu (Yang), has nourishing Yin and active Yang qualities within it. The dual unit of Yin/Yang exists within all life. For example, the Heart System stores Shen—that's a Yin function—but it also rules Xue—that's a Yang function. This characteristic association with either Yin or Yang and with both Yin and Yang is true of each Organ System—and of Yin and Yang itself, which is the unity of opposites.

THE ZANG (YIN) ORGANS

The Kidney System manages fluid metabolism, which the West associates with the kidneys and the adrenal glands. In addition, however, the Kidney System is responsible for storing surplus Qi. The Kidney System also rules birth, maturation, reproduction, growth, and regeneration.

The bones, inner ear, teeth, and lower back are also associated with the Kidney System, as is regulation of the growth of bone, marrow, and the brain.

The Kidney System stores Jing, and it provides it to other Organ Systems and body tissue. Also, the Kidney System is the root of eight important Channels that connect the Organ Systems to one another.

The Kidney opens up to the external world through the ear. Kidney harmony is revealed through acuity of hearing.

The Spleen System creates and controls Xue, as it is involved with the blood in Western medicine. It is also responsible for extracting Gu (Grain) Qi and fluids from food, transforming these substances into Ying (Nutritive) Qi and Xue, and storing Qi that is acquired by the body after birth.

The Spleen System also maintains the proper movement of ingested fluids and food throughout the body. The Spleen System transmits the Gu Qi upward and the pure fluids to the Lung and Heart Systems. Balanced fluid movement lubricates the tissues and joints. This prevents excess dryness, and it keeps fluids from pooling or stagnating and creating Dampness (see page 41). The Spleen likes dryness, and it is negatively affected by Dampness. The Spleen System also is associated with muscle mass and tone and with keeping the internal organs in place.

When the Spleen is balanced, the transformation and transportation of fluids is harmonious, Qi and Xue permeate the whole body, and the digestive tract functions well. The Spleen System's connection to the external world is through the mouth, and the Spleen's vigor is mirrored in the color of the lips.

The Liver System stores the Xue, and it is responsible for the proper movement of Qi and Xue throughout the body. It regulates the secretion of bile to aid digestion, balances emotions, and stores Xue. You can think of the Liver System as a holding tank where the Xue retreats when you are at rest. The Liver System also nourishes the eyes, tendons, and nails. The Liver System opens up to the world through the eyes, and its health is reflected in the sharpness of eyesight.

"The dual unit of Yin/Yang exists within all life."

The Lung System rules Qi by inhaling the Kong (Air) Qi from outside of the body, which, along with Gu and Yuan (Original) Qi, forms Zheng (Normal) Qi. As in Western medicine, the Lung System administers respiration, but it also regulates water passage to the Kidney System, which stores pure fluids. The Lung System also disperses water vapor throughout the body, especially to the skin, where it is associated with perspiration. In addition, the Lung System is in charge of Zong (Ancestral) Qi, which gathers in the chest, providing the Heart System with Qi. It also rules the exterior of the body through its relationship with Wei (Protective) Qi, providing resistance to External Pernicious Influences. (See "The Six Pernicious Influences" on page 40.) The nose is the gateway of the Lung System, and the health of the Lung System is reflected in the skin.

The Heart System is associated with the heart, the movement of the Xue through the vessels, and the storing of Shen. It is the ruler of the Xue and the blood vessels. When the Heart's Xue and Qi are in harmony, the Shen is at peace, and a person has an easy time dealing with what the world dishes out. The emotional states of joy, lack of joy, and charisma are associated with the Heart.

The Heart opens into the tongue, and abundant Heart Xue is revealed by moist and supple facial skin.

The Pericardium System is considered by some to be a distinct Organ System because it disperses Excess Qi from the Heart and directs it to a point in the center of the palm where it can exit the body naturally. The Pericardium is the protector of the heart muscle, and it provides the outermost defense of the Heart against external causes of disharmony. Although the Pericardium has no physiological function separate from the Heart, it has its own acupuncture Channel.

THE FU (YANG) ORGANS

The Fu Organs' main purposes are to receive food, absorb usable nutrition, and excrete waste. Fu Organs are considered less internal than the Zang Organs because they are associated with impure substances: food, urine, and feces. The Fu Organs and Channels can play a major role in acupuncture. The Fu Organs are the Gallbladder System, Stomach System, Small Intestine System, Large Intestine System, Urinary Bladder System, and the Triple Burner System.

The Gallbladder System works with the Liver System to store and secrete bile into the Large Intestine and Small Intestine Systems to help digestion. Any disharmony of the Liver System impacts the Gallbladder System, and vice versa.

The Stomach System receives and decomposes food so the Spleen System can transform the fluids and food essence into Qi and Xue. The Stomach System is also responsible for moving Qi downward and sending waste to the Intestines. Harmony between the Stomach and Spleen is vital.

The Small Intestine System works with the Stomach System to help produce Qi and Xue. The Small Intestine separates and refines the pure from the impure in fluids and food and in the mind.

The Large Intestine System moves the impure waste down through the body, extracting water and producing feces.

The Urinary Bladder System excretes urine, which is produced by the Kidney and Lung Systems and from intestinal wastewater.

The Triple Burner System is divided into three parts—the Upper Burner, Middle Burner, and Lower Burner—and does not exist in Western medicine. In Chinese texts, it is called San Jiao, and it is said to have a "name without shape." The best way to understand the Triple Burner is to examine its function, which is to mediate the body's water metabolism. Don't worry about where it lives, but seek to understand what it does.

- The Upper Burner is identified in the ancient Chinese text *Ling Shu* as an all-pervasive, light fog that distributes the Qi of water and food throughout the body. This part of the Triple Burner is associated with the head and chest and the Heart and Lung Organ Systems.

- The Middle Burner, identified as a froth of bubbles, is associated with the Spleen, Stomach, and sometimes the Liver. It's involved with digesting food, absorbing Essential Substances, evaporating fluids, and imbuing Xue with Nutritive Qi. The froth of bubbles refers to the state of decomposing, digested foods.

- The Lower Burner, which is called a drainage ditch, designates an area below the navel and includes the Kidney, Large and Small Intestines, Urinary Bladder, and Liver—due to the location of the acupuncture Channel. It governs the elimination of impurities. The Lower Burner helps regulate the Large Intestine System, and it helps the Kidney System process waste.

THE EXTRAORDINARY ORGANS

The Marrow, Bones, Brain, Uterus, Blood Vessels, and Gallbladder are called the Extraordinary Organs. The ancient Chinese medical text *Nei Jing* states that they resemble the Fu (Yang) organs in form and the Zang (Yin) organs in function.

Marrow and Bones: The Marrow, which includes the spinal cord, bone, and brain, are wedded to the Kidney System, and their existence depends on Jing, which gives rise to Brain and Marrow. The Marrow nourishes the bones.

The Brain is the Sea of Marrow. Consciousness is also associated with the Brain. The five senses, plus memory and thinking, are associated with other Organ Systems, but they are influenced by the Brain. Although the Heart stores the Shen, the Brain is also associated with it.

The Uterus, called *Bao Gong* (palace of the child), usually functions as a storage organ. However, in relation to menstruation and labor, its function is to discharge. While the Uterus is the anatomical source of menstruation and the location of gestation, its functioning is governed by other Organ Systems.

Both the Conception (Ren) and Penetrating (Chong) Channels (see page 31) arise from the Uterus. Menstruation depends on these Channels' harmonious functioning, on the strength of the Kidney Jing, and on the Xue functions of the Spleen and Liver Systems. Kidney Qi dominates the Uterus's reproductive function because reproduction is related to the Kidney. When the functions of the Heart, Liver, Spleen, and Kidney Systems are balanced, menstruation is normal. When the Heart and Kidney functions are strong, conception is easy.

Men are said to possess the energetic area of the Uterus. It contributes to their harmony, and it affects the flow of Essential Substances through the Conception and Penetrating Channels.

The Blood Vessels transport most of the Xue through the body. Although the distinction between Xue circulating in the Blood Vessels and in the Channels is not delineated, it's generally accepted that Blood Vessels carry more Xue, and Channels carry more Qi.

Understanding how the Blood Vessels function cannot be separated from understanding the relationship between the Xue and the Zang Organ Systems. Heart rules the Xue, keeping the heartbeat regular and balanced; the Liver stores and regulates the Xue, keeping an even flow of Xue throughout the body; and the Spleen governs the Xue, keeping it within the Blood Vessels and Channels. Disharmony of the Blood Vessels may be corrected by treating one of these Organ Systems.

The Gallbladder is considered both a Fu Organ and an Extraordinary Organ because it contributes to the breakdown of impure food—a Yang function—but unlike any other Yang Organ, it contains a pure fluid, bile.

"The Channels are a great aqueduct system that transports the Essential Substances to every part of the body."

The Channels

The Channels, sometimes called meridians or vessels, are
a great aqueduct system that transports the Essential
Substances—Qi, Jing, Xue, Jin-Ye, and Shen—to each Organ
System and to every part of the body. By tuning in to the way
Qi moves through the body's Channels, Chinese medicine
practitioners can "read" the harmony or disharmony of the
body's Essential Substances and Organ Systems. Practitioners
can also manipulate the flow of Qi and other Essential
Substances through the Channels to keep the flow irrigating
the body evenly.

Acupuncture (see chapter 5) controls the flow of the
Essential Substances by needling acupuncture points that
are positioned along the network of Channels like a series
of gates. At these points, the flow of Essential Substances,
particularly Qi, comes close to the surface of the skin,
and the needling stimulates or retards their passage
through the Channels.

According to Traditional Chinese Medicine (TCM), the functions of the Channels are to:

• Transport Xue and Qi and regulate Yin and Yang.

• Resist pathogens and reflect symptoms and signs of disease and disharmony.

• Transmit curative sensations that occur during acupuncture, such as the spreading of warmth and relaxation through the body, the sense of Qi moving, and a feeling of concentrated heaviness.

• Regulate Excess and Deficiency conditions.

The major Channels are divided into the Twelve Primary Channels, the Eight Extraordinary Channels, and the Fifteen Collaterals.

THE TWELVE PRIMARY CHANNELS

Each Primary Channel is linked to an Organ System, transports Qi and other Essential Substances, and helps maintain harmony in mind/body/spirit. The *Ling Shu*, part of the ancient Chinese medicine text, the *Nei Jing*, explains, "Internally, the twelve regular meridians connect with the Zang-Fu organs and externally with the joints, limbs, and other superficial tissues of the body."

The Twelve Primary Channels are Lung, Large Intestine, Stomach, Spleen, Heart, Small Intestine, Urinary Bladder, Kidney, Pericardium, Triple Burner, Gallbladder, and Liver.

Each Channel is defined by whether it starts or ends at the hand or foot, whether the Channel is Yin (runs along the center of the body) or Yang (runs along the sides of the body), and whether it is related to a Zang Organ System or a Fu Organ System.

The Cyclical Flow of Qi in the Twelve Regular Channels

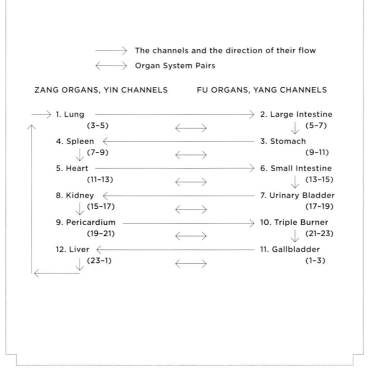

→ The channels and the direction of their flow

⟷ Organ System Pairs

ZANG ORGANS, YIN CHANNELS   FU ORGANS, YANG CHANNELS

1. Lung ——————————→ 2. Large Intestine
   (3–5)   ⟷   (5–7)

4. Spleen ⟵——————————— 3. Stomach
   (7–9)   ⟷   (9–11)

5. Heart ——————————→ 6. Small Intestine
   (11–13)   ⟷   (13–15)

8. Kidney ⟵——————————— 7. Urinary Bladder
   (15–17)   ⟷   (17–19)

9. Pericardium ——————————→ 10. Triple Burner
   (19–21)   ⟷   (21–23)

12. Liver ⟵——————————— 11. Gallbladder
   (23–1)   ⟷   (1–3)

Each Yin Channel and Zang Organ is paired with a Yang Channel and a Fu Organ. This association means that if one of the paired Organs becomes unbalanced, the other one may be thrown into disharmony as well.

The Stomach Channel of Foot—Yangming

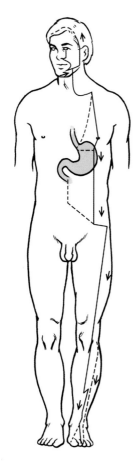

Yang Channel   ———
Internal Yang Channel   - - - - - - - -
Yin Meridian   ———
Internal Yin Channel   - - - - - - - -

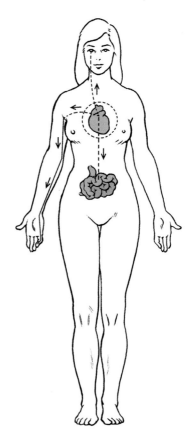

The Heart Channel of Hand—Shaoyin

THE EIGHT EXTRAORDINARY CHANNELS

In addition to the Twelve Primary Channels, there are Eight Extraordinary Channels. According to another ancient medical text, the *Nan Jing*, "The twelve organ-related Qi Channels constitute rivers, and the eight extraordinary vessels (channels) constitute reservoirs." Unlike the Twelve Primary Channels, the Eight Extraordinary Channels aren't associated with any of the twelve Organ Systems. But they are extremely important because they augment the communication between the Twelve Primary Channels, act as a storage system for Qi, and exert a strong effect on personality. These reservoirs collect Excess Qi, releasing it into the various Twelve Primary Channels if they become Qi Deficient because of mental or physical stress or trauma. They also have their own special functions.

Four of the Extraordinary Channels are located in the trunk of the body. They are solitary, unpaired Channels with special functions. They are the Chong Mai, the Ren Mai, the Du Mai, and the Dai Mai.

The Chong Mai (*chong-my*), or Penetrating Channel, is known as the Sea of Qi and Xue. It regulates the Qi and Xue of the Twelve Primary Channels and distributes Jing throughout the body. It brings the Kidney Qi upward to the abdomen and chest. The Chong Mai is the root of the other Extraordinary Channels.

The Ren Mai (*ren-my*), or Conception Channel, regulates the six Yin Channels and Yin throughout the body. It's in charge of the Jin-Ye and Jing, and it regulates the supply of body fluids to the fetus. Along with the Chong Mai, this Channel originates in the Uterus, supporting and supplying the Uterus.

The Urinary Bladder Channel of Foot—Taiyang

The Liver Channel of Foot—Jueyin

The Gallbladder Channel of Foot—Shaoyang

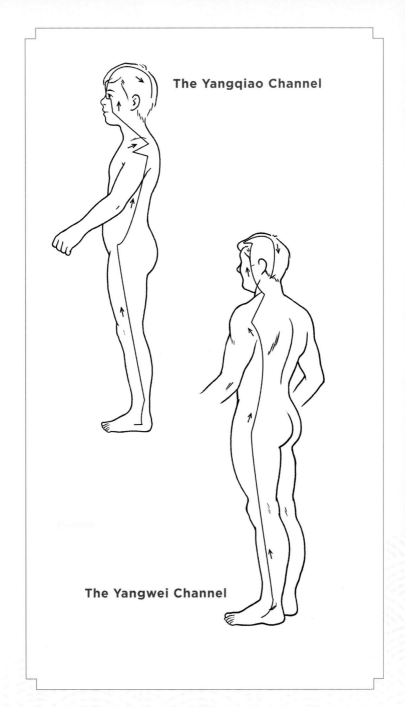

The Yangqiao Channel

The Yangwei Channel

The Du Mai (*doo-my*), or Governing Channel, also rises from the Uterus and links the Spinal Cord and the Brain and all of the Yang Channels. The Du Mai is the master of all of the Yang energy. Along with the Ren Mai, it regulates the balance of Yin/Yang, which in turn regulates the balance of Qi and Xue.

The Dai Mai (*die-my*), or Belt Channel, encircles the middle of the body like a belt. It links together all of the other Channels. It controls the Chong, Ren, and Du Mai, and it strengthens their links to the Uterus.

The last four Extraordinary Channels are located in the trunk and legs and are paired.

The Yangqiao Mai (*yang-chow-my*), or Yang Heel Channel, connects with the Governing Vessel. The Qi supplying this Channel is generated through leg exercises, and it rises upward to nourish the Yang Channels.

The Yinqiao Mai (*yin-chow-my*), or Yin Heel Channel, connects with the Kidney Channel. Qi enters the Channel through the transformation of Kidney Jing into Qi.

The Yangwei Mai (*yang-way-my*), or Yang Linking Channel, regulates Qi in the Yang Channels, including the Du Mai. Yangwei connects and networks the Exterior Yang of the whole body.

The Yinwei Mai (*yin-way-my*), or Yin Linking Channel, connects with the Kidney, Liver, and Spleen Yin Channels, the Ren Mai, and the Interior Yin of the whole body.

THE FIFTEEN COLLATERALS

These are branches of the Twelve Primary Channels. They run from side to side along the exterior of the body, and they have the same acupuncture points and names as the Twelve Primary Channels, plus the Du Mai, the Ren Mai, and the Great Collateral of the Spleen.

The Fifteen Collaterals are responsible for controlling, joining, storing, and regulating the Qi and Xue of each of the Twelve Primary Channels.

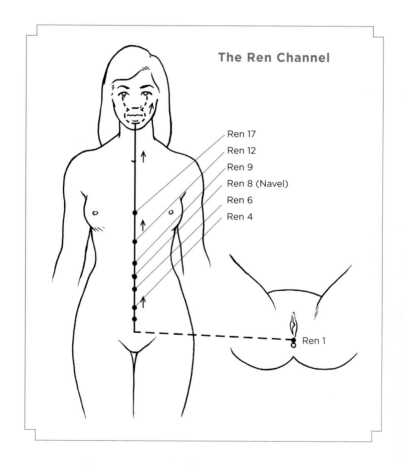

The Ren Channel

Ren 17
Ren 12
Ren 9
Ren 8 (Navel)
Ren 6
Ren 4
Ren 1

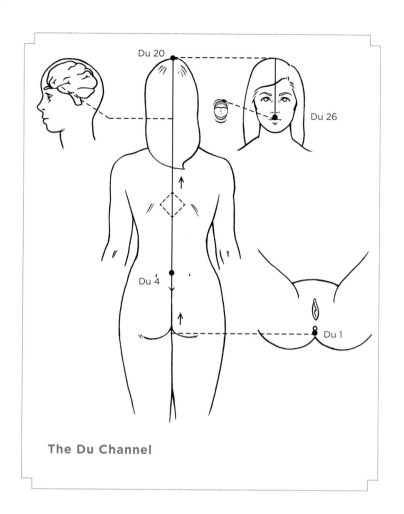

The Du Channel

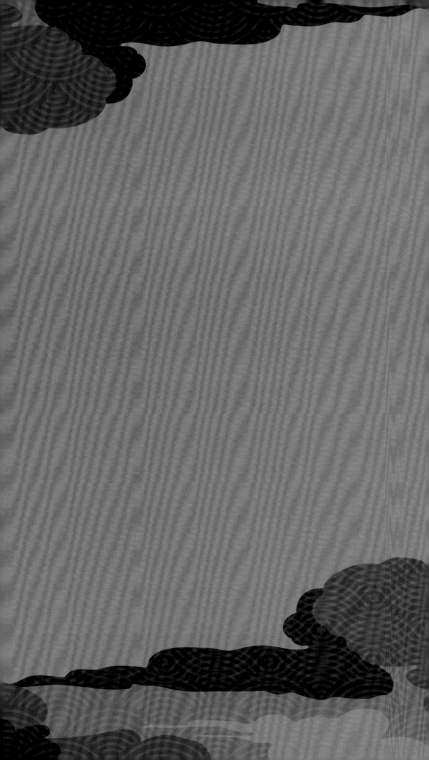

CHAPTER 2

CAUSES OF DISHARMONY AND DISEASE

A ncient Chinese medicine does not talk about viruses or bacteria as triggers of disease or disorders. Instead, it talks about influences, which cause disharmony in Yin/Yang, the Essential Substances, the Organ Systems, and the Channels.

Several categories of influences produce disharmony. Here, we will talk about two of the most important: the Six Pernicious Influences and the Seven Emotions.

The Six Pernicious Influences

The Six Pernicious Influences—Cold, Heat, Dampness, Dryness, Summer Heat, and Wind—are external climatic forces that can invade the body and create disharmony in the mind/body/spirit.

COLD

When hypothermia hits a skier or a mountain climber, muscle control fades, motion becomes slow and awkward, fatigue sets in, and the body shuts down. That's the same effect that the Cold Pernicious Influence has. It saps the body's energy, and it makes movements cumbersome. The tongue becomes pale; the pulse is slow. A person may develop a fear of cold and feel like sleeping in a curled-up position. Cold is Yin. If there's pain, it's eased by warmth.

When External Cold attacks the body, acute illness may develop, along with chills, fever, and body aches. When the External Cold moves inward and becomes an Interior Cold disharmony, it is associated with a chronic condition that produces a pale face, lethargy and grogginess, a craving for heat, and sleeping for longer than usual periods of time.

HEAT

Heat disorders feel like you've been playing tennis for two hours in the blazing sun. You're weary, and at the same time, you feel strangely cranked up. You can't stop talking about the game, but your words stick in your mouth. You won't feel like yourself again until you cool down and quench your thirst.

Heat disorders cause overactive Yang functions or insufficient Yin functions. They are generally associated with bodily heat, a red face, hyperactivity and talkativeness, fever, thirst for cold liquids, and a rapid pulse. Symptoms include carbuncles and boils, dry mouth, and thirst. Confused speech and delirium arise when Heat attacks the Shen.

DAMPNESS

Think about what happens to your backyard when it rains for two days. It becomes soggy, and water collects in stagnant pools. That is how Dampness affects the body. Damp pain is heavy and expansive, blocks the flow of Qi, and causes a stuffy chest and abdomen.

When External Dampness invades, it enters the Channels and causes stiff joints and heavy limbs. When Dampness invades the Spleen, it can cause an upset stomach, nausea, lack of appetite, a swollen abdomen, and diarrhea.

Interior Dampness—caused by either the penetration of External Dampness to the Interior or by a breakdown in the Spleen's transformation of fluids—may transform into Phlegm, which in Chinese medicine is more than simply a bodily secretion. It can cause obstructions and produce tumors and coughing. If Phlegm, also known as Severe Dampness, invades the Shen, it can lead to erratic behavior and insanity. Once Dampness has taken root, it is hard to displace.

DRYNESS

Dryness is a frequent partner with Heat. Think about the cracked bottom of a dried-up riverbed. But where Heat creates redness and warmth, Dryness creates evaporation and dehydration. External Dryness invading the body may create respiratory problems, such as asthmatic breathing and a dry cough, acute pain, and fever.

SUMMER HEAT

Summer Heat feels like the humid, oppressive weather that creates the dog days of August. It attacks the body after exposure to extreme heat and causes a sudden high fever and total lethargy. It is an External Influence and often arises with Dampness.

WIND

Wind animates the body, stirring it from repose into motion just as wind moves the leaves of a tree. When Wind enters the body, it is usually joined to another influence, such as Cold or Dampness.

If the body is infiltrated by Wind, the first symptoms usually appear on the skin, in the lungs, or on the face. Tics, twitches, fear of drafts, headaches, and a stuffed-up nose are symptoms.

When External Wind invades the body more deeply or when Wind arises due to internal problems, it is identified as Internal Wind. This can be associated with seizures, ringing in the ears, and dizziness.

STAGES OF HEAT- AND COLD-INDUCED PATTERNS OF DISHARMONY

When Heat or Cold invade the body, they create stages of disharmony. The symptoms associated with these stages help in the process of diagnosis and treatment. (Remember, Chinese medicine is not linear. These stages can appear in any order, or not at all.)

When there is a Cold invasion, it may pass through the following six stages:

- **Taiyang** (*tie-yang*) is characterized by cold, fever, headache, a stiff neck, and what is called a floating pulse.

- **Yangming** (*yang-ming*) is characterized by fever, no fear of cold/aversion to heat, irritability, thirst, possible digestive symptom such as fullness and constipation, and a full pulse. This is a stage of Interior Heat disharmony because Cold induces Heat in both the first and the second stages.

- **Shaoyang** (*shau-yang*) is characterized by malaria-like alteration of cold and fever, no appetite, a bitter taste in the mouth, tenderness along the sides, the urge to vomit, and a wiry pulse.

- **Taiyin** (*tie-yin*) is characterized by vomiting, loss of appetite, pain, and diarrhea, but no thirst. This is associated with a Deficient Spleen System.

- **Shaoyin** (*shau-yin*) is characterized by profound sleepiness, cold, and a weak pulse. Fever disappears. This is associated with Deficient Yang of the Kidney System. Rarely, it is associated with Yin Deficient Heat conditions.

- **Jueyin** (*zh-way-yin*) is characterized by upper body Heat and lower body Cold. When a Heat-induced disharmony moves into the body, it may pass in some order through one or more of the following four stages:

  - **The Wei** (*way*) **stage:** The body's natural defenses are attacked, and the result may be fever, slight fear of cold, coughing, headache, a reddish tongue, and a quick floating pulse.

  - **The Qi** (*chee*) **stage:** The Pernicious Influence penetrates the protective defenses of the body. The main symptom is usually high fever without chills, but symptoms vary, depending on which Organ System is affected. For example, Lung Heat produces high fever and coughing, while Stomach Heat produces high fever, abdominal pain, and constipation.

  - **The Ying** (*ying*)**stage:** Deeper penetration by Pernicious Heat increases the disharmony in mind/body/spirit. The symptoms of this stage include a bright red tongue, an easily disturbed spirit, restlessness or even mania, a rapid pulse, dark yellow urine, less thirstiness than in the Qi stage, and possible skin eruptions.

  - **The Xue** (*sch-whey*) **stage:** In the fourth and deepest stage, the Pernicious Influence of Heat enters the Xue (Blood), exacerbating the Ying-stage symptoms. Severe rashes, skin eruptions, high fever, and even coma may result. Blood in the urine or vomit may appear. Heat can injure the Yin, producing symptoms such as low fever, hot palms, dry teeth, a thin pulse, and stiffness and unresponsiveness.

EVALUATION OF THE TONGUE

The tongue is the mirror of the body. Harmony and disharmony are reflected in your tongue's color, moisture, size, coating, and the location of abnormalities.

A healthy tongue, is pinkish red, neither too dry nor too wet, fits perfectly within your mouth, moves freely, and has a thin white coating.

When examining your tongue, the Chinese medicine doctor looks at the color of the tongue body, its size and shape, locations of abnormalities, moistness or dryness, presence or absence of tongue fur, and the color and thickness of the coating or fur. These signs reveal overall state of health, and they also correlate to specific Organ System functions and disharmonies.

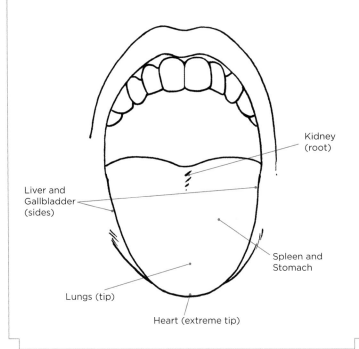

The Seven Emotions

While the Six Pernicious Influences are generally external triggers of disharmony, the Seven Emotions—Joy, Anger, Fear, Fright, Sadness, Grief, and Pensiveness/Worry—are internal causes of disease.

An Excess or a Deficiency of any emotion is indicative of disharmony in the mind and spirit, and it alerts the Chinese medicine practitioner to disharmonies in Organ Systems as well. The Heart and Liver are the most susceptible to emotions. The Heart stores the Shen, and unharmonious emotions can disturb the Shen and cause sleeplessness, muddled thinking, inappropriate crying or laughing, and, in extreme cases, fits, madness, and hysteria. Excess or Deficient Joy especially impacts the Heart.

The Liver, which is responsible for all of the emotions, is associated with anger. If the Liver Qi is stuck or in disharmony, the emotions become suppressed. If the emotions become suppressed, they suppress the function of the Liver. Sadness and grief, which are associated but distinct states, take their toll on the Lung System. If a person worries or overthinks, the Spleen System will become unbalanced. Fear and fright, which are also related but distinct emotions, interfere with the smooth functioning of the Kidney System.

The Eight Fundamental Patterns

The Eight Fundamental Patterns, which are paired as Interior, Exterior; Heat, Cold; Excess, Deficiency; and Yin, Yang, describe the way in which the External Pernicious Influences and the Seven Emotions create disharmony in the mind/

body/spirit. They also reveal the dynamic association of complementary yet opposed forces (Yin/Yang) within the body that have been thrown off balance by the presence of an influence or other disharmony.

Interior and Exterior patterns tell the practitioner where the disease resides. Interior patterns of disharmony are indicated if the disharmony is chronic, if it produces changes in the urine and stool, if there is discomfort or pain in the torso, and if there is no aversion to Cold or Wind. Exterior patterns of disharmony often come on suddenly and are acute. Common signs include chills, fever, a dislike of cold, and an achy feeling overall.

Heat and Cold describe the activity of the body and the nature of the disease. Deficient Yang or an External Pernicious Cold Influence causes Cold Patterns. Heat Patterns are caused by invasion of an External Pernicious Heat Influence, the Depletion of Yin substances, as well as Excess Yang.

Excess and Deficiency express the impact of the disharmony on the body's resistance to disease (Normal Qi). With Deficiency, there is underactivity in the Organ System(s), weakness and tentative movement, a pale or ashen face, sweating, incontinence, shallow breathing, and pain that is relieved by pressure. Excess is associated with overactivity of bodily functions; heavy, forceful movements; a loud, full voice; heavy breathing; and pain increased by pressure.

Yin and Yang encompass the other six Fundamental Patterns. Yin encompasses Interior, Cold, and Deficient. Yang encompasses Exterior, Heat, and Excess. To determine Yin/Yang disharmony, the doctor searches for clues about whether your disharmony is Interior or Exterior, for clues about patterns of Heat and Cold, and for clues about patterns of Deficiency and Excess. These can be translated into clinical symptoms.

After we examine the effect of the Eight Pernicious Influences and the Seven Emotions and the patterns of disharmony, the next step is for us to explore the pathologies of the Essential Substances, Organ Systems, and Channels. This will demonstrate how these lead to disharmony, the ways disharmonies manifest themselves, and how disharmonies affect the mind/body/spirit.

Disharmonies of the Essential Substances

QI DISHARMONIES

When Qi moves harmoniously throughout the body, there is wholeness and good health. When Qi is disrupted, disharmony and illness can arise. Unbalanced Qi may become Excess, Rebellious, Deficient, or Sinking or Collapsed.

Excess Qi almost always collects and pools and becomes Stagnant. Excess Qi and Stagnant Qi are associated with blockages in the Channels and Organ Systems. These blockages interfere with the circulation of Qi and cause it to pool up, deprive some areas of the body, and flood other areas. The blockages may occur due to suppressed emotions, External Pernicious Influences, poor diet, or traumatic injury. Symptoms of Excess and Stagnant Qi are pain that worsens with pressure and is not easy to pinpoint. You may ache all over and have trouble sitting still. Often the pain waxes and wanes, and it is related to your emotional state.

When Stagnant Qi becomes more severe, it may actually reverse direction and become **Rebellious Qi**. This disharmony causes vomiting, belching, hiccups, coughing, asthma, liver disturbances, and fainting.

Deficient Qi occurs when bad diet, lack of exercise, respiration problems, and/or disharmony of the spirit and mind use up Qi and don't replenish it. It can trigger spontaneous sweating, fatigue, weakness, lack of a desire to move, a weak voice, a pale but bright face, disharmony of a particular Organ System, and symptoms that become worse when you exert yourself. Deficient Qi is relatively Yin.

If the condition worsens or the Deficient Qi is left unchecked, it may become **Sinking or Collapsed Qi**. Sinking or Collapsed Qi is associated with organ prolapses (when it sags or falls down), dizziness, lack of stamina, and a bright, pale face.

SHEN DISHARMONIES

Shen disharmonies are usually triggered by an imbalance of the Seven Emotions. They are often accompanied by Stagnant Qi (often found in depression) and disharmony of the Heart and Liver Systems.

Disturbed Shen causes forgetfulness, disorientation, memory lapses, insomnia, and lackluster eyes. Extreme disharmony is associated with madness.

Lack of Shen is associated with a flat affect and inability to communicate. The classic phrase "The lights are on, but no one's home" describes this state.

To a Chinese medicine doctor, it makes no sense to heal the corporeal body without healing the Shen. The physical and spiritual are inseparable parts of the human being. Disharmony in your Shen is often the first hint of developing disharmonies and disease. Feeling out of sorts, fatigued, blue, grumpy, and dispirited may indicate that an illness is developing. If the practitioner and the client intercede early, when Shen is only mildly unbalanced, the development of full-blown disorders and disease may be forestalled.

XUE DISHARMONIES

Deficient Xue is associated with malnutrition, loss of blood, Deficient Spleen, depletion of Qi, and emotional stress. It can trigger insomnia, dry skin, dizziness, hair loss, palpitations, menstrual irregularities, and blurry vision. When there is Deficient Xue, your body doesn't receive sufficient nourishment, often in one or more Organ Systems. When the whole body is Deficient in Xue, your skin has a pallor and is dry.

  Excess or Stagnant Xue (also called Xue Stasis) is either caused by direct damage to the body's tissues (such as falling while skateboarding) or is a result of Stagnant Qi, Deficient Xue, and Cold Obstructing Xue. Symptoms include sharp, stabbing, fixed pain; tumors; or swollen organs. Pregnancy is a unique time in which an increase in Xue and Jin-Ye is part of a normal healthy body and is not necessarily associated with an Excess disharmony.

JING DISHARMONIES

We are born with Jing, and we can either deplete or replenish it throughout our lives. It always tends toward Deficiency. **Deficient Jing** symptoms include congenital disabilities, improper maturation, premature aging, sexual problems, and infertility. Disharmony of Jing is associated with Deficient Kidney.

JIN-YE DISHARMONIES

Deficient Jin-Ye is associated with dry lips, hair, eyes, and skin. **Excess Jin-Ye** is related to accumulation of fluids and produces edema and swelling.

The Effects of Disharmony on the Organ Systems

When External and Internal Pernicious Influences create disharmony, they upset the balance within and between each Organ System and the various Channels. Each Organ System has its own patterns of disharmony and associated symptoms.

DISHARMONIES IN THE ZANG (YIN) ORGAN SYSTEMS

Each of the Zang (Yin) Organ Systems can experience disharmony.

Kidney System

When the Kidney System becomes imbalanced, it may have one of four patterns of disharmony:

Deficient Kidney System Yang is associated with impotence, hearing loss, and incontinence. It is often associated with cold limbs, lack of Shen, swollen limbs, profuse clear urine, sore lower back, and loose teeth.

Deficient Kidney System Qi may trigger frequent urination, incontinence, bed-wetting, asthmatic breathing, and low back pain.

Deficient Kidney System Yin is associated with hot palms and soles, dry mouth, thirst, constipation, red cheeks, afternoon fevers, night sweats, insomnia, ringing in the ears, premature ejaculation, forgetfulness, and low back pain.

Deficient Kidney System Jing may lead to infertility, premature aging, retarded growth, lack or retardation of initial menstrual periods, and stiff joints.

Such disruptions are often associated with the emotional state of Fear and with the exercise of (or lack of ability to exercise) will.

Spleen System

Spleen System disharmony in general manifests in loose stools, abdominal fullness and distention, nausea, and poor appetite. Anxiety and the inability to concentrate are also associated with Spleen System imbalance. Congenital weakness, malnutrition, chronic diseases, and excessive mental activity are caused by Interior Spleen disharmonies.

Deficient Spleen System Qi symptoms are loose stools, poor appetite, abdominal distention and pain, pale complexion, fatigue and lethargy, weight gain due to fluid retention, edema, shortness of breath, and a pale bright face.

Sinking Spleen System Qi is a subset of Deficient Spleen Qi. Muscular weakness and prolapsed organs—particularly of the uterus, bladder, and rectum—characterize this disharmony.

Spleen System Not Able to Govern the Xue, another subset of Deficient Spleen Qi, is associated with Xue circulating outside its proper pathways. The symptoms are chronic bleeding such as bloody stools, nosebleeds, varicose veins, hemorrhoids, excessive menstrual bleeding, non-menstrual uterine bleeding, easy bruising, and purpura—purple spotting indicative of bleeding beneath the skin.

Deficient Spleen System Qi Leading to Dampness is a Deficiency condition leading to Excess.

Deficient Spleen System Yang develops from chronic Deficient Spleen Qi and Cold. The symptoms are the same as for Deficient Spleen Qi, plus clear copious urine, cold extremities and body, edema, weak digestion, and the desire for hot beverages.

Deficient Spleen System Yin appears in end-stage, life-threatening illness, such as AIDS and diabetes without the benefit of insulin. The symptoms include severe dryness, especially of the skin and lips, unquenchable thirst, loss of lean muscle mass, and severe wasting. Fever appears every afternoon and often in the evenings.

Externally caused Excess Spleen System patterns are often a result of an underlying Deficient Spleen System condition:

- Damp-Cold occurs when Spleen Yang becomes trapped by exposure to excessive Dampness. This can happen if you are being drenched by rain, wade through cold water, or are exposed to damp and cold temperatures for a prolonged time. The associated symptoms are lack of appetite, watery stools, fatigue, no thirst, and a lusterless, yellow face.

- Damp-Heat occurs when External Dampness and Heat invade the body or when Deficient Spleen System Qi leads to Excess Damp and combines with Heat. It results in the slowing of bodily functions, and it causes an accumulation of fluids. The symptoms are lack of appetite, a feeling of fullness in the stomach, fatigue, and scanty, dark urine. Sometimes it is associated with thirst without the desire to drink, itchy skin, and fever. It may also be associated with acute viral hepatitis.

Liver System

Repression of emotions is the most frequent cause of Liver System problems, which can manifest themselves in various patterns.

Stagnant Liver System Qi is the most common and usually the first Liver System disorder to appear when the system becomes imbalanced. It is an Excess condition, and it is relatively Yang. The main causes of Stagnant Liver Qi are emotional suppression and trauma. This leads to depression, uncomfortable feelings, and discomfort and pain between the ribs and in the chest, breast, and diaphragm. There may also be abdominal distention, restlessness, premenstrual congestion or distention, and a quick temper.

Stagnant Liver System Xue is characterized by fixed, sharp, stabbing pains and palpable masses. It often develops from Stagnant Liver Qi as well as Deficient Xue. In women, it is associated with missed menstrual periods, menstrual clotting and cramps, or severe trauma. In men, this pattern's appearance is almost always the result of severe trauma or severe illness.

Liver System Yang (or Fire) Rising develops when Stagnant Liver System Qi becomes more congested and severe. It is associated with an accumulation of Heat. Symptoms include headaches, eye pain, red eyes, sharp chest pain, scanty yellow urine, vertigo, nosebleeds, fits of anger, and dry stools. If left unchecked, this pattern can develop into a more serious condition—**Interior Liver System Wind**—that is associated with strokes, high fever with convulsions, paralysis, and loss of consciousness.

Deficient Liver System Xue is characterized by general dryness without any Heat symptoms. The symptoms are dry eyes and nails, blurry vision, dizziness, muscle spasms, reduced menstrual periods, twitching, and a pale, lusterless face.

Deficient Liver System Yin includes all of the symptoms of Deficient Liver System Xue, plus red cheeks and eyes, restlessness, hot flashes, headaches, dizziness, numb limbs, night sweats, dry mouth and throat, ringing in the ears, and a quick temper.

Damp-Heat of Liver System can occur when the diet is of poor quality and food is heavily spiced and fatty. It can also result from invasion of an Epidemic Factor, which is now known as viral hepatitis. The symptoms are discomfort in the top of the shoulders and rib cage, a bitter taste in the mouth, poor appetite, jaundice, fever and chills, and scanty, dark urine. Damp-Heat of the Liver System is associated with hepatitis and inflammation of the gallbladder.

Cold Obstructing the Liver Channel tends to be a male disharmony. Symptoms include a swollen scrotum and distention in the groin that is relieved by warmth.

Deficient Liver System Qi is rare. It creates Deficient Qi in the whole body, leading to a breakdown in joint function, general lethargy, shallow breathing, a lack of forcefulness in voice, and spontaneous sweating.

Lung System

General symptoms of Lung System disharmonies include dry skin or skin eruptions, shortness of breath on exertion, cough, asthma, allergies, nose and throat disorders, low resistance to External Pernicious Influences, and reduced energy.

Exterior Excess Lung System patterns include:

- Wind Cold is associated with chills, head and body aches, a lack of sweating, and frothy, thin, clear or white phlegm.

- Wind Heat is associated with fever, slight chills, sore throat, some sweating, a coarse cough, and thick, yellow, sticky phlegm.

- Wind Dryness is associated with a fever with chills, headache, dry throat and nose, and scant, dry phlegm.

Patterns of the Interior Excess Lung System include:

- Dampness is generally triggered by a pre-existing lack of Spleen and Kidney function. It is associated with a full, high-pitched cough, chest inflammation, difficulty breathing when lying down, wheezing, copious phlegm, no thirst, and a swollen face.

- Heat is generally triggered by overactive Liver and Heart Systems or the penetration of an External Pernicious Influence. When the Liver Invading the Lung causes it, the symptoms are dryness, pain in the chest or ribs, chest distention, and choking cough with thick green phlegm. When the Heart System causes it, the symptoms are insomnia, restlessness, cough, agitation, and confusion. When caused by an External Pernicious Influence, the symptoms are fever, sweating, cough, shortness of breath, and a rapid, superficial pulse.

Deficient Lung System patterns include the following:

Deficient Lung System Qi appears when the External Excess Pernicious Influence remains in the Lung and injures the Qi or when there are other Interior disharmonies that affect the Lung. The symptoms include a whispering voice, reluctance to speak, weak respiration, susceptibility to colds, weak cough, spontaneous sweating, shortness of breath that is worse with exertion, lack of warmth, and thin white phlegm.

Deficient Lung System Yin is associated with Deficient Jin-Ye of the Lung. The causes are Internal Dryness, chronic Deficient Kidney Yin, and the External Pernicious Influence of Heat remaining in the Lung and causing Dryness. Symptoms are fatigue; weakness; dry cough with no phlegm; restlessness; insomnia; afternoon fevers; night sweats; dry mouth and throat; weak voice; red cheeks; varicose veins; a feverish sensation in the palms, soles, and chest (Five Centers Heat); and sometimes scanty phlegm, streaked with blood.

Heart System

Deficiency patterns of the Heart System include:

Deficient Heart System Xue is often associated with Deficient Spleen Qi, because the Spleen is responsible for making the Xue. The symptoms include a pale lusterless face, dizziness, anxiety, confusion, excessive crying or laughing, and difficulty falling asleep.

Deficient Heart System Yin includes the symptoms of Deficient Heart Xue plus Heat symptoms, such as palpitations, agitation, insomnia, waking up at night, warm palms and soles, emotional lability, increased dreams, poor memory, night sweats, and physical and emotional hypersensitivity. It is often associated with Deficient Kidney Yin.

Deficient Heart System Qi is associated with the physiological problems of circulation, such as irregular pulse, arrhythmia, shortness of breath, fatigue, edema, and heart failure. Symptoms become worse with exercise.

Deficient Heart System Yang includes the symptoms of Deficient Heart Qi plus Cold symptoms, such as pain and distention in the chest, cold limbs and/or coldness throughout the whole body, purplish lips, and a slower, weaker heartbeat. It often appears with Deficient Kidney Yang and Deficient Lung Qi.

A subset of Deficient Heart System Yang is **Collapse of Yang**, in which Yin and Yang can separate, and the person is near death. Symptoms include profuse sweating, extremely cold limbs, purple lips, and confusion.

Patterns diagnosed as Excess include:

Excess Heart System Fire is caused by extreme emotional excitement, sunstroke, or excess consumption of hot, pungent foods, drinks, or herbs. Symptoms include insomnia, restlessness, red face, inflammation or soreness of the tongue and mouth, thirst, and scanty, burning urine with blood.

Excess Phlegm Obstructing Heart System or Misting of the Orifices may arise from Spleen Dampness or simply from a general internal lack of proper fluid circulation. The symptoms include Shen disharmony, aberrations of consciousness, coma or semi-coma, excessive weeping or laughing, depression or dullness, mania, incoherent speech, muttering to oneself, drooling, and predisposition to stroke.

There are two types of Phlegm: **Excess Cold Phlegm** symptoms are a withdrawn, inward manner;

muttering; staring at walls; and sudden blackouts. **Excess Hot Phlegm** symptoms include hyperactivity, agitation, aggression, incessant talking, and violent lashing-out behavior.

Heart System Stagnant Qi is associated with a stuffy chest and difficulty breathing. If it is the result of Stagnant Phlegm, there are the same symptoms plus excess phlegm expectoration, abdominal fullness, nausea, and vomiting.

Heart System Stagnant Xue is associated with angina and pectoral pain, and it results from Deficient Heart Qi or Deficient Heart Yang. Symptoms include palpitations, shortness of breath, irregular pulse, fixed stabbing pain, and a purple face.

Pericardium System

Only one major pattern is associated with the Pericardium System, and it is not an independent pattern: **Excess Phlegm Obstructing Heart System or Misting of the Orifices** (see page 59).

DISHARMONIES IN THE FU (YANG) ORGAN SYSTEMS

Each of the Fu (Yang) Organ Systems also can experience disharmony.

Stomach System

The patterns of disharmony that may afflict the Stomach include the following.

Food Retention in Stomach System is due to irregular eating habits, overeating, or eating hard-to-digest foods. Retention blocks passage of Qi in the abdomen, triggering distention, fullness, and pain in the abdomen; foul belching;

regurgitation; anorexia; vomiting; and difficult bowel movements.

Retention of Fluid in Stomach System Due to Cold is associated with a constitutional Deficiency of Stomach and Spleen Qi, complicated by the invasion of the External Pernicious Influence of Cold. Eating too much cold or raw food can trigger this pattern. Symptoms include fullness and pain in the stomach relieved by warmth, reflux of clear fluid, or vomiting after eating. This pattern is associated with prolonged disease.

Hyperactivity of Fire in Stomach System (also called **Stomach Heat**) may arise from eating too many hot, fatty foods and from depression. The symptoms include burning and pain in the stomach, thirst for cold beverages, bleeding gums, and scant, yellow urine. It's often associated with stomach ulcers, excessive appetite, constipation, and mouth ulcers.

Deficient Stomach System Yin occurs when hyperactivity of Fire in the Stomach consumes the Stomach Yin or when Stomach Jin-Ye dries up because of persistent Heat due to a prolonged disease with fever. Symptoms include burning stomach pain, hunger without appetite, dry heaves, hiccups, dry mouth and throat, constipation, and an empty, uncomfortable feeling in the stomach.

Triple Burner System

Damp-Heat in the Upper Burner can happen when Damp invades the body and stays in the muscles and upper body, damaging Spleen Qi. Symptoms include extreme dislike of cold, mild or no fever, feeling like there is a soft band around the head, heavy arms and legs, a feeling that an elephant is standing on your chest, lack of thirst, distended abdomen, noisy bowels, loose stools, and lack of facial expression.

Damp-Heat in the Middle Burner can arise from the External Pernicious Influences of Summer Heat and Damp. It can also occur when Damp-Heat from the Upper Burner sinks into the Middle Burner. Poor nutrition is also a trigger. Symptoms are similar to those for invasion of Damp and Heat in the Stomach and Spleen: heavy arms, legs, and trunk; full, distended chest and stomach; nausea; vomiting; anorexia; loose but difficult stools; dark urine; feeling thirsty with little desire to drink; and a fever that can't be felt at the first touch of the skin but that becomes evident after the skin is felt for a rather long time. In severe cases, the Shen is disturbed, and mental abilities are affected.

Damp-Heat in the Lower Burner affects the Intestine Systems and Urinary Bladder System. It is associated with difficulties with urination and elimination. Symptoms include constipation, thirstiness with little inclination to drink, and a hard, distended lower abdomen.

Gallbladder System

Disharmony with the Gallbladder System manifests similar to disharmony with the Liver System, specifically **Liver Damp-Heat**. The symptoms associated with that pattern include discomfort in the chest, a bitter taste in the mouth, poor appetite, fever and chills, jaundice, and scanty, dark urine. General Gallbladder dysfunction can cause you to become angry and impulsive, along with an inability to make up your mind and exhibiting general weakness of character.

Small Intestine System

Pain Due to Disturbance of Small Intestine System Qi may result from poor nutrition, carrying overly heavy loads, and wearing clothing that's inappropriate for the weather, making you vulnerable to External Pernicious Influences. Symptoms include acute lower abdominal pain, abdominal distention, noisy bowels, and a heavy, downward-pushing sensation in the testes accompanied by lower back pain.

Heart Fire Moving to the Small Intestine System includes the symptoms of Heart Fire (see "Excess Heart System Fire" on page 59), plus irritability, cold sores, sore throat, frequent painful urination, and a full feeling in your lower abdomen.

Large Intestine System

Large Intestine System Damp-Heat is sometimes called **Damp-Heat Dysentery**. This pattern often occurs in hot climates in the summer and autumn when the External Pernicious Influences of Summer Heat, Dampness, and Toxic Heat invade the Stomach and Intestines. It also arises when a person eats too much raw, cold, or unsanitary food or eats at irregular times. Symptoms include abdominal pain, a feeling of urgency along with difficult bowel movements, watery diarrhea, bloody stools with mucus, burning anus, and dark-colored urine. Sometimes it is accompanied by fever and thirst.

Consumption of Jin-Ye of Large Intestine System is often seen in the elderly, after childbirth, and in the later stages of disease with fever. Symptoms include constipation, dry stools, and dry mouth and throat.

Intestinal Abscess is known in Western medicine as appendicitis. The symptoms include acute pain in the lower right quadrant, aversion to touch, and possibly a fever.

Urinary Bladder System

Damp-Heat in the Urinary Bladder System is the main pattern of disharmony associated with the Urinary Bladder System. This pattern can arise from the invasion of External Pernicious Damp and Heat or from a diet of excessively hot, greasy, and sweet foods. Symptoms include painful, frequent, urgent urination; cloudy, dark urine; back pain; blood in the urine; feeling of fullness in the lower abdomen; burning pain in the urethra; and difficult urination.

DISHARMONIES OF THE EXTRAORDINARY ORGANS

Each of the Extraordinary Organs—the Marrow and Brain and Uterus—also can experience disharmony.

Marrow and Brain

When the Marrow is Deficient, the Brain becomes unbalanced. Symptoms include ringing in the ears, vertigo, shakiness, poor eyesight, and difficulty thinking. Weak bones and retarded bone growth can also occur.

Uterus

If there is Deficient Heart Xue, the Heart Qi does not descend to the Uterus, and the menstrual periods may become irregular or stop. Failure of Kidney Jing to descend to the Uterus can result in infertility, irregular periods, or complete cessation of menstruation. Disturbances of the Extraordinary Channels, such as the Chong Mai and Ren Mai (which arise in the Uterus), can also cause Uterus disharmonies.

Because of the interdependence of the Uterus on other Organ Systems and Channels, treatment for all menstrual and reproductive problems is through the Liver, Kidney, Spleen, or Heart Organ System and related Primary and Extraordinary Channels.

The Effects of Disharmony on the Channels

Channels are affected by disharmonies that are distinct from those afflicting Organ Systems and the Essential Substances. Some practitioners who solely practice acupuncture will primarily diagnose and devise treatments through the diagnosis of Channel disharmonies.

When a pathogen causes disharmony in a Channel, the acupuncture points become tender to the touch. These spots are useful in diagnosis because they clue the practitioner to the location and nature of the imbalance along the Channel and in the associated Organ System(s).

The following are the pathologies identified by the TCM school of thought that correspond to the Twelve Primary Channels, Eight Extraordinary Channels, and Fifteen Collaterals. (Not all schools of acupuncture accept these indications for diagnosis and treatment, however.)

PATHOLOGIES OF THE TWELVE PRIMARY CHANNELS

Each of the Twelve Primary Channels is associated with distinct disharmonies. These disharmonies, which arise when the flow of Qi is disrupted, create symptoms in the part of the body through which the Channel flows. Each Channel has exterior and interior pathways. The exterior pathways are relatively near the surface of the skin while the interior pathways are relatively deep and cannot be needled directly.

DISHARMONIES OF THE TWELVE PRIMARY CHANNELS

CHANNEL	STAGE	SYMPTOMS
Lung Channel of Hand	Taiyin	cough, asthmatic breathing, coughing up blood, congested and sore throat, the feeling that a baby elephant is standing on your chest, pain in the neck, pain in the upper chest, pain running along the lower section of the inside of the arm
The Large Intestine Channel of Hand	Yangming	nosebleeds, runny nose, toothaches, congested and sore throat, neck pain, pain in the front of the shoulder and the front edge of the arm, noisy bowels, abdominal pain, diarrhea, dysentery
The Stomach Channel of Foot	Yangming	noisy bowels, distended abdomen, edema, vomiting and stomach pain, hunger, bloody nose, a droopy mouth, congested and sore throat, chest and abdominal pain, pain along the outside of the leg, fever, mania
The Spleen Channel of Foot	Taiyin	belching, vomiting, stomach pain, distended abdomen, loose stools, jaundice, overall feeling of lethargy and heaviness, inflexibility and pain where the tongue attaches to the mouth, swelling and cold along the inside of the knee and thigh

CHANNEL	STAGE	SYMPTOMS
The Heart Channel of Hand	Shaoyin	heart pain, palpitations, chest and rib pain, insomnia, night sweats, dry throat and thirst, hot palms, pain along the inside of the upper arm
Small Intestine Channel of Hand	Taiyang	deafness, yellowing of the whites of the eyes, sore throat, swollen cheeks and throat, pain along the back edge of the shoulder and arm, lower abdomen distention and pain
Urinary Bladder Channel of Foot	Taiyang	bed-wetting or trouble urinating, depression and mania, blocked and stuffy nose, teary eyes (particularly in the wind), runny nose, eye pain, bloody nose, headache, pain along the Urinary Bladder Channel from the nape of the neck to the middle of the backs of the legs
The Kidney Channel of Foot	Shaoyin	bed-wetting, too-frequent urination, nocturnal emission, impotence, asthmatic breathing, coughing up blood, dry tongue, congested and sore throat, edema, lower back pain, irregular periods, pain along the back edges of the insides of the thighs, weak legs, hot soles of the feet

CHANNEL	STAGE	SYMPTOMS
Pericardium Channel of Hand	Jueyin	heart pain, palpitations, tight chest and trouble breathing, emotional restlessness, depression and mania, flush face, swelling in the armpits, arm spasms, hot palms
The Triple Burner (Sanjiao) of Hand	Shaoyang	distended abdomen, bed-wetting, painful urination, deafness, ringing in the ears, pain at the outer edge of the eyes, swollen cheeks, congested and sore throat, pain behind the ears, shoulder pain, and pain in the backs of the arms and elbows
The Gallbladder Channel of Foot	Shaoyang	headache, pain at the outer edges of the eyes, jaw pain, blurry vision, a bitter taste in the mouth, swelling and pain in the upper chest and armpits, pain along the outside of the chest and rib area, pain in the outsides of the thighs and lower legs
The Liver Channel of Foot	Jueyin	low back pain, fullness in the chest, pain in the lower epigastric area, hernia, pain on the top of the head, dry throat, hiccups, bed-wetting, painful urination, mental disharmony

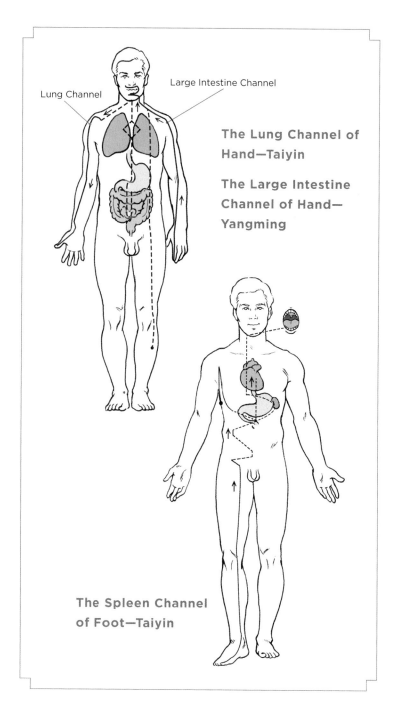

Lung Channel

Large Intestine Channel

The Lung Channel of Hand—Taiyin

The Large Intestine Channel of Hand—Yangming

The Spleen Channel of Foot—Taiyin

The Gallbladder Channel of Foot—Shaoyang

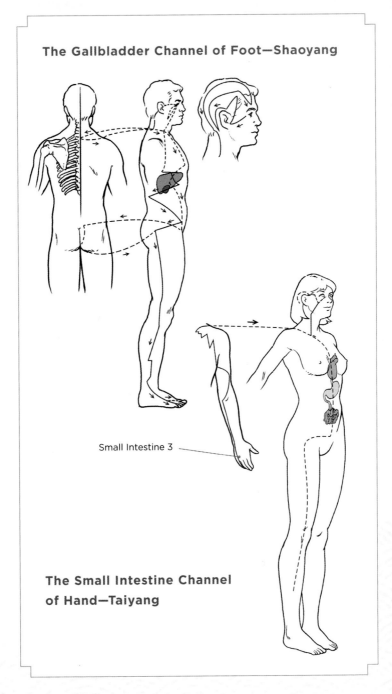

Small Intestine 3

The Small Intestine Channel of Hand—Taiyang

PATHOLOGIES OF THE
EIGHT EXTRAORDINARY CHANNELS

These Channels are closely related to the Liver System, Kidney System, Uterus, and Brain and Marrow, and they serve to connect the Twelve Primary Channels and regulate their Qi and Xue. The pathological manifestations in this chart are based on the physiological functions and the area of each Channel's influence. You can work with them during self-massage and acupressure. These Channels have a big role in disharmonies of women's reproductive cycles.

DISHARMONIES OF THE EIGHT EXTRAORDINARY CHANNELS

CHANNEL	SYMPTOMS
Du Mai (Governing Channel)	stiff, painful spine; severe muscle spasm causing arching of the back; headache; epilepsy
Ren Mai (Conception Channel)	vaginal discharge, irregular periods, infertility in women and men, hernia, nocturnal emission, bed-wetting, urinary retention, stomach pain, lower abdominal pain, genital pain
Chong Mai (Penetrating Channel)	spasm and pain in the abdomen, irregular periods, asthmatic breathing, infertility in women and men, emotional and physical problems arising from various forms of abuse
Dai Mai (Belt Channel)	weak lower back, vaginal discharge, uterine prolapse, trouble moving the hips and legs, weakness and muscular atrophy of lower limbs, an unaccountable feeling like one is sitting in water

CHANNEL	SYMPTOMS
Yangqiao Mai (Yang Heel Channel)	insomnia, redness and pain at the inside corners of the eyes, pain in the back and lower back, turning out of the foot, spasm of the lower limbs, epilepsy
Yinqiao Mai (Yin Heel Channel)	epilepsy, lethargy, leg spasms, turning in of the foot, lower abdomen and lower back pain, hip pain that causes referred pain in the pubic region
Yangwei Mai (Yang Linking Channel)	External symptoms, such as chills and fever
Yinwei Mai (Yin Linking Channel)	Internal symptoms, such as chest and heart pain and stomachaches

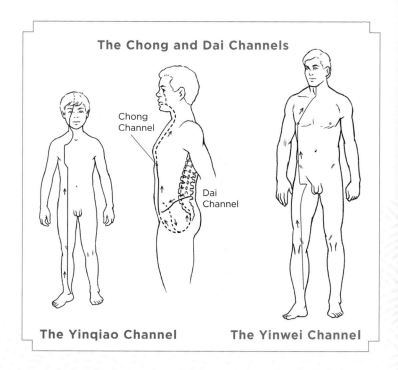

The Chong and Dai Channels

Chong Channel

Dai Channel

The Yinqiao Channel   **The Yinwei Channel**

PATHOLOGIES OF THE FIFTEEN COLLATERALS

The Fifteen Collaterals branch off of the Primary Channels with which they are associated. They strengthen the relationships between the paired Channels, and they move Qi and Xue to organs and tissue in the body. When disharmony occurs, the Collaterals compound the symptoms of the Primary Channel with which they are associated.

DISHARMONIES OF THE FIFTEEN COLLATERALS

COLLATERAL OF THE ...	STAGE	SYMPTOMS
Lung Channel of Hand	Taiyin	hot palms and wrists, shortness of breath, bed-wetting, frequent urination
Intestine Channel of Hand	Yangming	toothache, deafness, cold teeth, a stifling feeling in the chest and diaphragm
Stomach Channel of Foot	Yangming	depression and mania, atrophy of muscles and weakness in the lower legs, congested and sore throat, sudden attacks of hoarseness
Spleen Channel of Foot	Taiyin	spasm of the abdomen, vomiting, diarrhea

COLLATERAL OF THE . . .	STAGE	SYMPTOMS
Heart Channel of Hand	Shaoyin	chest and diaphragm fullness, aphasia
Small Intestine Channel of Hand	Taiyang	weak joints, muscular atrophy, impaired movement in the elbows, skin warts
Urinary Bladder Channel of Foot	Taiyang	stuffed-up sinuses, runny nose, headache, back pain, bloody nose
Kidney Channel of Foot	Shaoyin	low back pain, urinary retention, mental restlessness, a stifling sensation in the chest
Pericardium Channel of Hand	Jueyin	heart pain, mental restlessness
Triple Burner (Sanjiao) of Hands	Shaoyang	flaccidity or spasm on the insides of the elbows
Gallbladder Channel of Foot	Shaoyang	cold feet, paralysis of the legs, inability to stand upright

COLLATERAL OF THE ...	STAGE	SYMPTOMS
Liver Channel of Foot	Jueyin	constant erection, itching in the pubic area, swollen testes, hernia
Ren Mai		abdominal pain that exerts an outward pressure, itching of the abdominal skin
Du Mai		stiff spine, heavy sensation in the head, head tremor
Great Collateral of the Spleen		overall achiness, muscle pain, weakness in the arms and leg joints

CHAPTER 3

DIETARY THERAPY

D iet, herbs, acupuncture, bodywork, and exercise/ meditation are the therapeutic tools of Chinese medicine. They are used to build, maintain, and restore wholeness in mind/body/spirit. Diet is extremely important because every day what you eat either nourishes or dilutes your Essential Substances.

There are four dietary principles of Chinese medicine dietary practices.

Dietary Principle One: You Are What You Eat—and What You Don't Eat

Food has tremendous powers in Chinese medicine—powers that extend far beyond the Western concept of food as fuel, providing calories, carbohydrates, protein, fat, vitamins, and minerals. These powers are defined as Food Energetics, which cool or warm the metabolism and Organ Systems, moisturize or dry the Organ Systems, and increase or decrease the flow of Qi, Jing, and Xue.

A healthy diet harnesses Food Energetics by combining foods that balance each other, so no one energetic influence becomes too strong.

Balance your Food Energetics. If your diet contains an imbalance of Food Energetics, your various Organ Systems and your Qi, Jing, Shen, and Xue are subjected to more of a drying than a moisturizing influence, or more of a cooling than a warming influence. This can cause Stagnation or Depletion of your Qi, Jing, and Xue and disharmony of Shen, making you vulnerable to diseases and discontent.

Don't eat too many raw foods. To balance Food Energetics, eat warm foods to keep the digestive process working well. Despite common beliefs, raw foods are not closer to nature, and they do not contain better nutrition. Chinese medicine sees raw foods as depleting. They may cause a Cold-Damp condition because your body has to expend extra energy to "cook" the food in your Stomach. The only people who should eat raw foods in higher than the recommended amounts are those who are very Hot.

Avoid iced and frozen foods. It takes warmth and Qi to digest foods that are cold, and this uses up the digestive Fire. Therefore, all foods should be warmed up and cooked if they are cold or frozen, such as frozen vegetables. You should only rarely eat ice cream or frozen yogurt. When you do, I often recommend drinking ginger tea first to warm up the digestion.

Chew each bite of food carefully. This makes the digestive process easier and conserves the digestive Fire. This Fire is produced by the Central Qi, which warms the central Organ Systems so they have the power to digest food. Cold food cools that inner warmth, and that's why it's not good to eat too many cold or raw foods.

Don't stuff yourself. Overeating overwhelms the digestive Fire and causes Stagnation and disease.

Drink scant liquid during meals. If you drink too much liquid during meals, you'll drown the digestive Fire.

Eat organic foods as much as possible. The elimination of synthetic pesticides, hormones, antibiotics, and other chemical residues in vegetables, meats, and dairy increases available Qi, removes antagonists to your overall health, and also makes food taste better. Today, with the proliferation of harmful chemical additives to food, we must add eating organic foods to the top of our list of most important dietary considerations.

If you eat meat, it is best to eat meat from animals that have been fed organic diets. For beef, it is best that the cows have been grass-fed for their entire lives. Researchers at California State University in Chico reviewed three decades of research and found that beef from grass-fed cows is lower in saturated fats, contains more omega-3 fatty acids and antioxidants, and is lower in calories.

Eat unprocessed foods as much as possible. Simply put, avoid eating foods that come out of boxes or bags. In particular, do not eat any foods with high fructose corn syrup (HFCS). Read every label because many foods have HFCS.

Dietary Principle Two: Most of Your Food Should Be Eaten in Season

Your diet should be dictated by the rhythms of the external world. Food gains power to maintain health from its relationship to the external world. Food, the fuel of the mind/body/spirit, should be taken into the body in a pattern that's attuned to the rhythms of the environment. This perspective is based on the Tao, the Chinese philosophy of the unity and interrelationship between the external and internal worlds.

As you look around the outside world, you can see that in the spring, energy moves up. In the summer, it moves out. In the fall, energy moves down, and in the winter, it moves inward. Likewise, green sprouting vegetables, such as lettuce and bean sprouts, move energy up, so enjoy more of them in the spring. Spices, flowers, and leaves, such as basil and edible flowers, have outward-moving energy, so enjoy plenty of them in the summer. Root vegetables, such as burdock and turnips, have downward-moving energy, so give in to the natural desire to eat them in the fall. Grains, seeds, and nuts, such as almonds and buckwheat, have inward-moving energy, so eat plenty of them all winter long.

To reap the benefits of food's energetic relationship to the seasons, you may want to eat foods in their own season when their power is strongest or in the season before to prepare your body for the coming season.

Dietary Principle Three:
Moderation and Variety in Diet Are Essential for a Balanced Mind/Body/Spirit

Understand the spirit of a balanced diet. A balanced diet results from a combination of the foods you eat and the way you prepare, eat, and think about your food. You could not create the perfect diet pill that combined all the Food Energetics needed to achieve wholeness and harmony. Food Energetics is not simply the result of chemistry. It is also a result of spiritual forces. The power of food—positive and negative—to influence your mind/body/spirit is affected by how it is prepared, served, and eaten.

There is no list of good foods and bad foods. Eating too much of a healthy food is unhealthy. For example, you can overdo broccoli and whole grains. Small amounts of unrefined sugars are not necessarily unhealthy. However, too much sugar or highly processed refined sugar or high fructose corn syrup is. Organic meats in small quantities may be useful in some people's diets. Eating too much meat or meat that is processed or containing chemicals is not healthy.

Balance comes from eating a wide variety of food, including vegetables, grains (especially low glycemic), fish, meats, fruits, and dairy, each in moderation. If you do that, you can pretty much eat most foods. The percentages of each type of food that you should eat depend upon your constitution and your specific Chinese medicine patterns.

The modern American diet notion that you should only eat from a roster of mildly unappealing, healthy foods and avoid all "bad" foods is not doable for many people. For example, if you have a little bit of chocolate, it is not a sin. In fact, we now know it may have good anti-inflammatory effects.

As important as moderation is in achieving balance, it is also vital to strive for the proper attitude toward food. Food prepared as a gift, served calmly, eaten with respect, and digested in a harmonious atmosphere bestows positive benefits. Food slapped together without regard or with resentment, served as quickly as possible, gobbled down, or eaten while driving, watching TV, or even reading cannot be assimilated healthfully.

Be flexible. It's so easy to get fanatic about diet. But rigidity about how you eat is itself a disease-producing behavior, even if you're being rigid about eating healthy foods. Health depends on a graceful adaptability to your surroundings and your ability to nourish yourself, even if perfect foods aren't available.

Dietary Principle Four:
Food Is Powerful Medicine

Chinese medicine's dietary practices form the basis for effective preventive medicine. When you eat foods that maintain the flow of Qi and the harmonious functioning of the Organ Systems, the immune system remains strong, bones and muscles remain flexible and supportive, digestion is good, the skin is healthy, the mind and spirit remain clear, and stress and anger dissipate.

However, the effect of diet on bodily functions is not linear, and it cannot be viewed as a process of cause and effect. Instead, the association between food, Qi, Jing, Shen, Xue, the Organ Systems, and digestion depends on each element's influence over and reaction to the other elements.

This feedback mechanism is reflected in the role of the Spleen and Stomach Systems, which govern digestion and the assimilation of food. The Stomach System releases the energy stored in food, and the Spleen System distributes the food energy through the body. This maintains a harmonious flow of Qi, which in turn helps nourish the Spleen and Stomach Systems with an ample supply of Essential Substances, keeping them in balance. Without a well-balanced diet, the entire network of interdependence is interrupted.

You can also see the delicate yet powerful interdependence of diet and healthy (or unhealthy) Organ Systems when you look at the relationship between diet and the Triple Burner System—particularly the Middle Burner.

Food keeps the Middle Burner balanced so it maintains a strong Middle Burner Fire, which allows for proper digestion. If the Fire becomes weak through lack of proper foods, the

Middle Burner is forced to supplement its Fire with energy drawn from the Lower Burner. When that happens, Kidney Fire, which the Lower Burner fuels, may become depleted. That, in turn, can cause anxiety, imbalance, or agitation in the mind and spirit. Agitation in the mind and spirit can interfere with proper digestion. Before you know it, you've become trapped in a cycle of depletion and disharmony affecting mind/body/spirit—all because your diet was not balanced and couldn't support the Middle Burner's Fire.

Correcting Disharmonies through Dietary Therapy

Chinese Dietary Therapy provides a powerful tool for correcting disharmonies, and it is used in conjunction with herbal therapy (see chapter 4), acupuncture (chapter 5), and Qi Gong (chapter 6) to restore balance to the Essential Substances, Organ Systems, and Twelve Channels. Generally, Diet Therapy can help sedate Excess, tonify Deficiency, cool Heat problems, warm Cold problems, moisten Dry problems, and dry Excess Dampness. *Symptoms* describe what you feel when you are not well. *Signs* are the manifestations of disharmony that Chinese medicine practitioners look to guide them in identifying and diagnosing particular imbalances.

DEFICIENT QI

Symptoms include lethargy, loose stools, fatigue, weakness, decreased appetite, shortness of breath, and occasionally cold extremities and frequent urination.

Signs include a thin, weak pulse and a tongue that is pale, possibly swollen with tooth marks.

"Without a well-balanced diet, the entire network of interdependence is interrupted."

Western diagnoses include chronic fatigue, asthma, and urinary incontinence.

Your diet should contain: Traditional Chinese theory says that half of total calories should come from grains and legumes, a third from vegetables, and about 15 percent from fish or meats. With meats, you don't want to tax your digestion or build Phlegm—so eat only about 2 to 3 ounces (55 to 85 g) of animal protein per serving. Five percent of total calories can come from dairy. Recommended foods include rice or barley, broth, leeks, string beans, sunflower seeds, and carrots. However, modern understanding of the glycemic index as well as protein intake gives us the ability to modify this diet. In this case, when one eats carbohydrates, it is best to eat low- to moderate-glycemic carbohydrates with a low glycemic load. It is important to eat these carbohydrates along with sufficient protein to balance the glycemic index and load.

Your diet should not contain: Raw food, salads, fruits, and juices in excess.

To treat cold symptoms with Deficient Qi: Add dried ginger, cinnamon bark, and chicken's eggs.

DEFICIENT SPLEEN QI

Symptoms include lack of appetite, bloating, mild abdominal pain better with pressure, loose stools, and fatigue.

Signs include a weak pulse and pale, soft tongue with tooth marks and thin white fur.

Western diagnoses include diarrhea, gastric or duodenal ulcers, anemia, and even chronic hepatitis.

Your diet should contain: Cooked, warming foods, such as squash, carrots, potatoes, rutabagas, turnips, leeks, onions, rice, small amounts of chicken, turkey, mutton or beef, cherries, strawberries, figs, cardamom, ginger, cinnamon, nutmeg, custards, and small amounts of honey, molasses, maple syrup, and sugar.

Food should be well chewed and eaten in moderate amounts.

Your diet should not contain: Salsa, citrus, too much salt, tofu, millet, buckwheat, milk, cheese, seaweed, and excess sugar.

DEFICIENT SPLEEN QI LEADING TO DEFICIENT YANG

If Deficient Spleen Qi is not treated early, the body becomes ever more depleted. The Qi cannot be replenished through what you eat and drink. Eventually, a more serious Yang Deficiency develops.

Symptoms include aversion to the cold, craving warm drinks, and chilled fingers, toes, ears, and nose tip.

Signs include a slow, thready pulse and tongue that is moist and pale with indentations/tooth marks on the sides.

Western diagnoses include swelling, gastritis, enteritis, kidney disease, and colitis.

Your diet should contain: Foods as noted for Deficient Spleen Qi (see page 87).

Your diet should not contain: Raw or chilled foods or foods that are difficult to digest, such as fatty foods, raw cruciferous vegetables, and milk.

DAMPNESS ASSOCIATED WITH DEFICIENT SPLEEN QI DEFICIENCY

This is a complicated case of Excess and Deficiency.

Symptoms include headaches, watery stools, and queasy stomach.

Signs include a slippery pulse, tongue fur that is thick and greasy, and a tongue body that is swollen with tooth marks along the sides.

Western diagnoses include hepatitis, dysentery, gastroenteritis, parasites, and severe diarrhea.

Your diet should contain: Foods as denoted for Deficient Spleen Qi (see page 87) along with foods that drain Excess Dampness, such as barley, corn, adzuki beans, garlic, mushrooms, mustard greens, chicken, alfalfa, shrimp, scallions, and rye.

Your diet should not contain: Too much red meat, salt, or sugar and food that produces Damp, including dairy products, pork, shark meat, eggs, sardines, octopus, coconut milk, cucumber, duck, goose, seaweed, olives, soybeans, tofu, spinach, pine nuts, and alcohol.

SPLEEN QI DEFICIENCY WITH DAMP-COLD

Symptoms include water retention, puffiness, feeling cold, mild nausea, trouble breathing, watery stools, and clear, frequent urine.

Signs include a pulse that is weak and slippery or soft and slow and a pale tongue with tooth marks on the sides.

Western diagnoses include edema, parasites, ulcers, and Crohn's disease.

Your diet should contain: The traditional recommendation of about 65 percent of total calorie intake from grains or legumes. Around 25 percent of your diet should be vegetables. Eat 10 percent red and white meat, with no more than 25 ounces (700 g) a week. Modern recommendations would lower the intake of carbohydrates to closer to 30 percent. Also, the wisdom is to eat low-glycemic carbohydrates in balance with high-quality proteins to lower the glycemic index as well as the glycemic load.

Your diet should not contain: Raw food, fruits, sugar, and dairy products.

SPLEEN DEFICIENCY WITH DAMP HEAT

Symptoms include a hot and heavy feeling, fever, nausea, costal or abdominal pain, labored breathing, and diarrhea.

Signs include a weak and slippery or soft pulse that's rapid and a tongue that's swollen and reddish, possibly with yellow fur.

Western diagnoses include colitis, acute hepatitis, and Crohn's disease.

Your diet should contain: The traditional diet of 65 to 70 percent of calories from grains and legumes, 25 to 30 percent from cooked vegetables, and 5 percent from white meats with not more than 6 to 12 ounces (170 to 335 g) in a week. An occasional salad is suggested.

Your diet should not contain: Red meat, raw vegetables (other than the occasional suggested salad), fruit juices, and dairy.

UPWARD MOVEMENT OF QI AND PHLEGM

This condition is the result of several underlying disharmonies that, only when added together, create symptoms. First, the stresses and strains of daily life coincide with a stressful diet of sugar, caffeine, and alcohol or drugs. This exhausts the Kidney Fire (in the Lower Burner), and digestion (Middle Burner) becomes sluggish. Phlegm builds up. Simultaneously, stress triggers an elevation in Liver Yang. Negative emotions make the Liver energy rise upward. Qi and fluids from the Lung rise and become rebellious and erratic. This combines with the Excess Phlegm production.

Symptoms include sexual problems, cold extremities, low back pain, susceptibility to every passing cold or flu, joint pain, fear, anxiety, and impatience.

Signs vary, but whatever else is present, there are all the signs of weak Spleen, Kidney, and Stomach Systems.

Western diagnoses include sinus allergies, watery eyes, skin rashes, sinus headaches, and chronic cough.

Your diet should contain: Cooked foods, rice, barley, mung beans, sweet rice congee, adzuki beans, mustard greens, and broth-based vegetable soups.

Your diet should not contain: Sugar, coffee, alcohol, citrus, dairy, soy, and all raw, iced, or chilled foods and all energetically Cool and Cold food.

EXCESS HEAT

Symptoms include warm or hot extremities, sweatiness, acne or boils, decreased bowel movements, a loud voice, irritability, and feeling hot.

Signs include a rapid, full pulse and a red tongue that may have a yellow coating.

Western diagnoses include skin disorders along with redness, digestive difficulties, chronic constipation, manic behavior, and/or headaches.

Your diet should contain: Almost half of total calories should be grains and legumes. A third should be cooked and raw vegetables. About 20 percent could be juices and fruits.

Your diet should not contain: Frozen or icy foods or chicken. Eat only minimal amounts of meat, sugar, and dairy products.

"Symptoms describe what you feel when you are not well. Signs are manifestations of disharmony."

STAGNANT LIVER QI

Symptoms include tenderness in the rib cage, nausea, premenstrual lability, irritability, and swollen breasts and abdomen.

Signs include a wiry pulse and a tongue that is dusky or purplish.

Western diagnoses include alcohol abuse, type A personality, fibrocystic breasts, swelling or lumps in groin or breasts, goiter, PMS, menstrual irregularities, hepatitis, and headaches.

Your diet should contain: Liver-sedating foods, such as beef, chicken livers, celery, kelp, mussels, nori, and amazake (a fermented rice drink). Also recommended are foods that regulate or move Qi, including basil, bay leaves, beets, black pepper, cabbages, coconut milk, garlic, leeks, peaches, and rosemary.

Your diet should not contain: Alcohol, coffee, fatty foods, fried foods, excessively spicy foods, excessive red meat, and sugar.

FLUID DRYNESS

Symptoms include dry throat, dizziness, emaciation, spontaneous sweating, and shortness of breath. Other symptoms vary, depending on whether the underlying syndrome is Deficient Xue or Deficient Yin.

Signs include a pulse that is fine, halting, or hollow and weak and a tongue that is uncoated and pink.

Western diagnoses include type 2 diabetes and chronic constipation.

Your diet should contain: Dairy products, most non-citrus fruits, honey, pork, liver congee, tofu, olive oil, peanut oil, and sesame oil. For Deficient Kidney Yin, eat kidney congee and liver congee. (See "Deficient Xue" below for additional guidelines.)

Your diet should not contain: Raw fruits and vegetables, cold foods, caffeine, purgative herbs and medicines, and alcohol.

Special note: If you have type 2 diabetes, combining a Chinese medicine diet along with incorporating an understanding of the glycemic index is incredibly important.

DEFICIENT XUE

Symptoms include dizziness, low weight, blurred vision, tingling in toes or fingers, dry skin or hair, and a pale, lusterless face. The symptoms vary, depending on the relative Deficient Xue.

Signs include a thready or hollow pulse and a pale tongue.

Western diagnoses include anemia; headaches; anxiety; nervousness; lack of, painful, or possibly heavy periods; dry skin; and dry constipation with difficult stools.

Your diet should contain: Oysters, sweet rice, liver, chicken soup, Dang Gui Chicken, eggs, and green beans.

Your diet should not contain: Raw fruit and vegetables, cold liquids, and ice.

STAGNANT XUE

Stagnant Xue results from a traumatic injury, as a manifestation of gynecological imbalances, and the outcome of long-term Stagnant Qi or Deficient Xue.

Symptoms include missed periods, excessive clotting with period, fixed painful lumps, dry skin and lips, thirst, susceptibility to cold extremities and constipation, and liver (or other organ) fibrosis.

Signs include a choppy pulse and a tongue that is purple and may have purple spots on the sides or on other parts, along with purple or blue sublingual veins.

Western diagnoses include endometriosis, menstrual cramps, pelvic inflammatory disease (PID), uterine fibroids, fibrosis/cirrhosis, bruising, and fixed pain.

Your diet should contain: A small amount of chives, cayenne, eggplant, saffron, safflower, basil, brown sugar, and chestnuts to improve circulation of the Xue.

Foods and spices that disperse Stagnant Xue include turmeric, adzuki beans, rice, chives, garlic, vinegar, basil, scallions, leeks, ginger, chestnuts, cayenne, nutmeg, eggplant, and white pepper.

Foods that strengthen the Stomach and Spleen Organ Systems to promote sufficient production of Xue include rice, trout, and small amounts of chicken and chicken liver.

Foods that build Yin, which strengthens Xue, include mussels, wheat germ, and millet.

Your diet should not contain: Duck, alcohol, fatty foods, and sweets. If you are cold, avoid citrus fruits and tomatoes.

CHAPTER 4

HERBAL THERAPY

In 3,500 BCE, Shen Nung, the god of husbandry, founded Chinese herbal medicine. According to a tale passed down through the ages, he had a hole in his stomach through which he watched his internal processes. Because of this remarkable ability, he became curious about what happened to his body when he ate various plants, minerals, and animals. This led him to take 365 types of herbs to determine their healing effects. But even a god could not dodge the perils of experimentation with unknown herbs. After cataloging hundreds of them, he died of poisoning. Here's a tip: Never take any herbs without consulting a trained herbalist.

Forms of Herbal Medicines

Chinese herbs come in many forms, such as bulk herbs, decoctions, powders, pills, syrups, plasters, pellets, medicinal wines, tinctures, and enemas. You can tell what form an herb will come in by its name. If it includes the word *tang*, it will be a decoction. *San* means it is a powder. *Wan* or *pian* indicates it is a pill.

Bulk herbs are generally processed before they are used in herbal therapy. They may be altered to detoxify components that would otherwise be harmful. Bulk herbs can be processed to change the way the herb works. Some examples of these processes are baking, dipping in honey, boiling, or frying the substance before it is turned into powders and decoctions.

Decoctions are made by cooking a combination of prepared bulk herbs in water to make an herb soup, which is sometimes called a tea. They are useful because, unlike pills, they can be individualized with each prescription.

Decoctions are particularly effective against acute problems, such as the External Pernicious Influences like Wind Cold. They are usually only prescribed for a few days. If the herbs are required for chronic conditions, many practitioners will provide pills or powders, although bulk herbs may be used as well.

Decoctions are also used for steaming, making poultices, and other external applications. Not all herbs should be made into decoctions, however. Some Fu Zheng herbs, such as ganoderma, which is in many immune-modulating formulas, are more effective in other forms.

HERB FORMS

You can tell what form an herb will come in by its name. The following italicized terms are the most common. You can find their descriptions below.

Pian = a pill

San = a powder

Tang = a decoction

Wan = a pill

Powders are created in two different ways. The first way is by pulverizing the bulk individual herbs or herb formula. The second way is by decocting, concentrating, and spray-drying the individual herb or formula and creating dry granules. Powders or granules are commonly swallowed with warm water either as a powder or in capsules. Sometimes the powders or granules are placed into boiling water in a Thermos and steeped overnight to create a tea. Practitioners may either put together individual formulas from single granulated herbs, or they may order and prescribe granules of prepared formulas. Often, a prepared formula is used as a base and individualized with single herbs.

Pills in the form of Chinese herbal tablets and capsules almost always contain herbal formulas rather than individual herbs, and they are targeted to treat specific disharmonies. There are different types of herbal pills. Some are made from powders, and others are made from concentrates. Practitioners and clients often favor pills over bulk herbs because they are less expensive and easier to use; they are formulated for specific disharmonies; they may have a more concentrated pharmacological effect; and they provide access to otherwise rare or expensive herbs.

Syrups are prepared by reducing herbs to a thick concentrate. Granulated sugar or honey is added, and the syrups are then ingested orally.

Plasters are made by preparing herbs in oil along with other substances. The resulting salve is spread over a cloth that is used as a compress or plaster or directly applied to the skin or orifice.

Pellets or special pills are usually made from extremely rare medicinals. They are super-refined into a fine powder that is mixed with a gluey substance. Pellets are used internally and externally.

Medicinal wines are therapeutic beverages made by soaking or simmering herbs in wine.

Tinctures or extracts are drinks or topical formulas made by steeping herbs in alcohol or glycerin.

Enemas are made from easily dissolved herbs or cooked teas and used to remedy digestive problems along with other internal conditions.

With the advent of modern manufacturing processes in China, in the tradition that everything always changes, new processes for manufacturing are continually being developed and used.

Choosing a Qualified Herbalist

Only a competent, trained herbalist should prescribe Chinese herbal remedies. Taking recommendations from untrained personnel at health food stores, through mail-order catalogs, or from untutored practitioners is foolish at best and dangerous at worst.

In my clinic, I try to buy from herbal companies that sell only to licensed, primary health care providers or licensed pharmacies.

Chinese herbal medicine is not a separately licensed profession; therefore, licensing is not required unless they also practice acupuncture in a state that licenses acupuncture. Most states do not require herbal training or examination for acupuncture licensure.

However, the National Certification Commission for Acupuncture and Oriental Medicine (NCCAOM) does provide certification through a national examination for Chinese herbal medicine. As of this writing, only nine states require the NCCAOM herbal examination for acupuncture licensure, but many practitioners are nationally certified. You can check on the NCCAOM website for specific details.

Some well-trained and qualified practitioners are not nationally certified. If you go to a Chinese herbalist who has been prescribing and/or dispensing herbs for years, of course it is best for you rely on personal recommendations and reputation as well as asking how he or she was trained in herbal medicine.

Regarding herbal quality assurance, to know the quality and testing of the herbs, practitioners can ask their herbal supplier for a certificate of analysis (COA) for the herbs that are sold to them.

SIDE EFFECTS OF HERBS

Some herbs and formulas, especially pills or granules, may cause undesirable side effects. The most common are digestive problems. This may result from the fact that pills and granules contain the natural plant fiber. People who do not get much fiber in their diets before taking herbs, herb pills, or granules find that the herbs may increase their fiber intake dramatically. These people might experience digestive side effects, such as gas and bloating. These effects usually pass after two to three days, as the body adjusts to increased fiber intake and begins to rebalance itself.

If side effects persist, often changing the time of day the herbs are ingested and/or their dosage can control them. Sometimes a digestive formula needs to be added to the herbal regimen to restore balance. A practitioner can tell the difference between the presence of a disease that causes digestive upset and herbal side effects.

An Herbal Sampler

The following chart is a sample of the individual herbs that I prescribe extensively in my clinic as part of herbal formulas. These herbs are commonly used in many Chinese medicine practices.

COMMON HERBS AND THEIR USES

HERB	CHARACTERISTICS
Astragalus membranaceus (*Huang Qi*)	• tonifies Spleen and Lung Qi • increases overall energy • aids in digestion and absorption of food • stops spontaneous sweating • promotes urination • helps heal injured tissue
Atractylodes alba or white atractylodes (*Bai Zhu*)	• tonifies the Spleen and Stomach • removes Spleen Dampness • helps with digestion, relieves edema, helps increase body weight and muscle strength • supports immune system • lowers blood sugar • prevents concentration of glycogen in the liver
Bupleurum root (*Chai Hu*)	• used to treat diseases that cannot be categorized as either Interior or Exterior, but that are in the process of moving inward • spreads Liver Qi • raises the Spleen Qi in order to harmonize Spleen and Stomach Deficiency patterns, reduce fever, and calm the mind

HERB	CHARACTERISTICS
Codonopsis (*Dang Shen*)	• strengthens and harmonizes the functions of the Spleen and Stomach • tonifies Qi, increases red blood cells, and enhances T-cell activity • used to overcome fatigue, reverse appetite loss, strengthen tired limbs, stop diarrhea, ease phlegmy cough, and support digestive functions • supports the Kidney and Lung Qi
Cordyceps (*Dong Chong Xia Cao*)	• used for extreme fatigue, tuberculosis, impotence, post-disease weakness, and spontaneous sweating • supports the Kidney and Lung Qi
Angelica sinensis (*Dang Gui*)	• tonifies and moves Xue • used for menstrual disorders • disperses cold • alleviates pain • moistens dry stools
Eclipta prostrata (*Mo Han Lian*)	• nourishes and tonifies the Liver and Kidney Yin • cools Xue • used as a liver-protecting compound for people with hepatitis and liver disease
Ganoderma (*Ling Zhi*)	• tonifies the Xue • calms the Spirit • used in asthma, insomnia, anxiety, and immune modulation, especially cancer support

A BIT ABOUT FU ZHENG

Today cordyceps is known as a Fu Zheng herb. *Fu Zheng* means "restore the normal" in Chinese. The Fu Zheng herbs encompass a number of herbs, such as ganoderma and astragalus. The Fu Zheng concept was fully developed in China during the 1970s to provide support for people undergoing Western cancer treatments, especially to support the immune system and strengthen Qi. More recently, in the 1980s, our group at Quan Yin Healing Arts Center in San Francisco, along with a few other Western practitioners, specifically adapted this approach to working with people with immune deficiency diseases, including people with HIV/AIDS.

A wealth of cell and animal studies and the early development of clinical trials support its use. Studies of cordyceps include research into liver fibrosis, for enhancement of chemotherapy in small-cell lung cancer through specific polysaccharides in cordyceps, along with compounds shown to kill human leukemia cells. In China alone, more than 100 institutes are devoted to the development of medicinal uses of fungi, including this ancient herb.

HERB	CHARACTERISTICS
Ginseng (*Ren Shen*), species *Panax ginseng*	• tonifies the Spleen and Lung • calms the Spirit • revitalizes Qi • used for insomnia, palpitations, and forgetfulness • effects on the central nervous system • acts as an antihistamine • affects the metabolism • is cardioprotective
American ginseng (*Xi Yang Shen*), species *Panax quinquefolium*	• replenishes the Yin and Qi • cools Fire from Deficient Yin • tonifies the Lung Yin • promotes the secretion of bodily fluids • reduces irritability • stops cough due to Deficient Lung Yin • stops night sweats • improves overall energy
Isatis leaf (*Da Qing Ye*) and isatis root (*Ban Lan Gen*)	• has antiviral and antibacterial properties • used for viral meningitis, pneumonia, and bacterial infections

HERB	CHARACTERISTICS
Licorice root (*Gan Cao*), also *glycyrrhiza*	• harmonizes herbal formulas • tonifies the Spleen Qi • moistens the Lung • removes toxins • drains Fire • used for fatigue and loose stools, to help remedy weak digestion, and to decrease effects of toxic substances • **Warning:** In prolonged high doses, licorice root may have a steroidal effect, causing high blood pressure, water retention, reduction in thyroid function, and decrease in the basal metabolic rate. When properly prescribed, very small amounts are used. Always take *glycyrrhiza*, especially in its extracted forms, under the care of a qualified, licensed health care provider.
San Qi	• disperses Xue and Qi • used for pain relief and to stop bleeding
Scutellaria (*Ban Zhi Lian*), species *Scutellaria barbata*	• invigorates Xue • promotes urination • reduces swelling and sores

HERB	CHARACTERISTICS
Spatholobus (*Ji Xue Teng*)	• vitalizes and tonifies Xue • used for menstrual pain, lack of menses, irregular menstruation, abdominal pain, numbness in the extremities, lower back pain, and knee pain • **Warning:** Spatholobus increases contractions in the uterus, so it's contraindicated during pregnancy unless specifically prescribed by a Chinese herbalist and your Western doctor.

CHAPTER 5

ACUPUNCTURE AND MOXIBUSTION

Classic acupuncture is the art of inserting fine, sterile, metal filiform needles into certain points along the Twelve Channels and Fifteen Collaterals (tributaries of the Channels) to control the flow of Qi. These days, practitioners also use electrostimulation of the needles, lasers, and even ultrasound to stimulate the points.

Moxibustion, the burning of the herb moxa (Chinese mugwort) over Twelve Channel points and certain areas of the body, is used to warm, tonify, and stimulate. It also induces the smooth flow of the Essential Substances, prevents diseases, and preserves health. Doing moxa regularly on specific acupuncture points is said to promote strength and longevity. In fact, an old Chinese saying is, "Never take a long journey with a person who does not have a moxa scar on [the acupuncture point called] Stomach 36." (It's important to note that moxibustion as it is generally used today does not cause scars. A particular type of moxa, called scarring moxa, was used by the ancient Chinese for longevity and stamina. Scarring moxa is not covered by our malpractice insurance today, but it is still used by some practitioners.)

Acupuncture

Acupuncture, as described traditionally, is the art and science of manipulating the flow of Qi and Xue through the body's Twelve Channels—the invisible aqueduct system that transports the Essential Substances to the Organ Systems, tissues, and bones. Manipulation of the Qi and Xue is accomplished by the stimulation of specific acupuncture points along the Channels where the Essential Substances flow close to the skin's surface.

Present-day practitioners use many different methods for stimulating acupuncture points, including electrostimulation and lasers as well as the traditional fine metal needles. Whatever the technique, acupuncture is relatively painless. It is often accompanied by feelings of heaviness or warmth and sensations of movement. These sensations occur because acupuncture points are like gates in an aqueduct system.

When the points are stimulated, they may open a gate, so that Excess or Stagnant Qi or Xue can disperse. Or if Qi and Xue are Deficient, stimulation of certain acupuncture points may close a gate, so the Essential Substances can collect as needed. When this is done, the distribution of Essential Substances throughout the whole system of Channels becomes more evenly balanced, allowing for a smoother flow into all areas of the body.

This adjustment of the body's Qi and Xue can be used to maintain or restore balance between Yin and Yang, alleviate emotional disorders, protect the Organ Systems, moisten tendons, and keep the joints healthy. Acupuncture works on a spiritual level and on a physical, energetic level.

TRADITIONAL CHINESE MEDICINE ACUPUNCTURE

As Charles Chace, a noted Chinese medicine scholar, pointed out in an article on the diversity of Chinese medicine, "While specific people throughout history may have believed they had a lock on the truth, the Chinese as a people never took this very seriously and never really strove toward a single truth. Chinese society as a whole never cared about a single truth. They just cared about what is useful, about what makes logical sense. . . . A concept of absolute knowledge is not Chinese, and also the concept of either/or is not Chinese. Chinese medicine has historically allowed opposing points of view to exist simultaneously."

TCM acupuncture is based on the Eight Fundamental Patterns, Seven Emotions, Essential Substances, Organ Systems, and Channels. There are 365 basic acupuncture points located along the Twelve Primary Channels, Eight Extraordinary Channels, and Fifteen Collaterals.

Whichever type of acupuncture you receive, it will be effective for diagnosis, prevention, and treatment of disharmony.

Diagnosis: When the body is in disharmony, acupuncture points along the Channels become tender to the touch, alerting the practitioner to the location of disturbances in the Channels and in associated Organ Systems. Some points become particularly tender when disease is present, and they offer vivid diagnostic help.

Prevention: Acupuncture maintains a balanced flow of Qi and Xue. By using it for regular tune-ups, you can keep your mind/body/spirit in harmony. Furthermore, acupuncture can be used to prevent disease from becoming more severe. You may have noticed emotional and spiritual changes or disturbances often appear as the first sign of illness and imbalance: You don't quite feel right, you might have dream-disturbed sleep, or you might become easily irritated. These early clues to the onset of disease can be present in the body, and they can be identified through careful diagnosis before symptoms emerge. Acupuncture can then be used to rebalance the Qi and prevent the developing disharmony from turning into a full-blown illness or disorder.

Treatment: In the TCM system of acupuncture, we adjust the flow of Essential Substances so that Excesses are dispersed, Deficiencies are overcome, Dampness is dispelled, Dryness is eased, Cold is warmed, and Heat is cooled. It reestablishes balance and promotes a self-healing response by stimulating communication pathways within the body that promote tissue repair and natural pain control.

Acupuncture—used alone or in conjunction with dietary therapy, herbal remedies, bodywork, and Qi Gong—is a powerful force for promoting health and well-being.

THE TAO OF ACUPUNCTURE

When a Chinese medicine practitioner uses acupuncture for diagnosis and treatment, he or she does not view the person's health as a phenomenon that is isolated from what is going on in the world outside or the general stages of life. Climate, geographic location, and age and individual conditions all impact the harmony of the mind/body/spirit. Consequently, they must be taken into consideration in evaluation and in the development of a treatment plan.

Climate

According to the ancient Chinese text *Ling Shu*, "In spring, the pathogenic factors are most likely to attack the superficial layer; in summer, they are most likely to attack the skin; in autumn, they are most likely to attack the muscles; and in winter, they are most likely to attack the bones and tendons." In treatment of such disorders, the *Ling Shu* also says that techniques should remain consistent with the seasons, "that's why in the spring and summer, shallow acupuncture is generally used, and in winter and autumn, deep acupuncture is preferred."

Geographic Location

Geographic location has an impact on acupuncture treatment because climate affects diet and lifestyle, which in turn affects the way Essential Substances and Organ Systems function.

Age and Individual Conditions

Acupuncture treatment is also tailored to the age, gender, and general constitution of the recipient. People of different ages and genders have different physiologies. The *Ling Shu* explains these distinctions: "A middle-aged strong person with sufficient Qi and Xue and hard skin may, if being attacked by pathogenic factors, be treated by a deep needling with a needle retained for some time. . . . An infant has weak muscles and less volume of Qi and Xue, [so] acupuncture treatment is given twice a day with shallow needling and weak stimulation." The text also suggests deep needling for people engaged in physical labor and shallow needling for people who perform mental work.

HOW DOES ACUPUNCTURE WORK?

While it is important scientifically to research the mechanisms of acupuncture, the science of how acupuncture works is not the primary basis on which a practitioner develops a treatment plan and uses acupuncture.

TCM describes acupuncture's impact on the mind/body/spirit in the following six ways:

Reinforcing is used when there are no strong pathogenic forces at work in the body. It bolsters the Organ Systems, and it replenishes Yin, Yang, Qi, and Xue.

Reducing dispels pathogenic factors and breaks up Stagnation. Reducing is used for Excess conditions.

Warming removes blockages in the Channels, nourishes Qi, dispels Cold, and restores Yang.

Clearing dispels Heat and remedies Heat syndromes with swift needling.

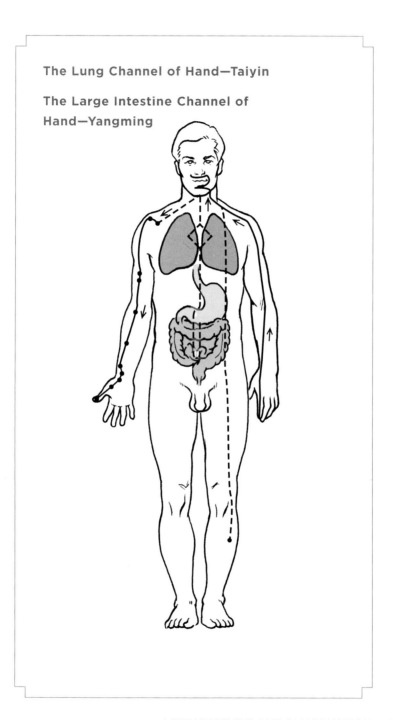

The Lung Channel of Hand—Taiyin

The Large Intestine Channel of
Hand—Yangming

The Triple Burner (Sanjiao)
Channel of Hand—Shaoyang

Triple Burner 15

Triple Burner 5

Triple Burner 4

back of right hand

Ascending raises Qi, prevents Sinking Qi, and prevents Organ prolapse.

Descending sends Upward Rebellious Qi downward and subdues Yang. It is not generally used when Deficiency is present. (Note: The difference between Sinking and Descending Qi is that Sinking indicates what happens to Qi when it is not being supported or helped up. Descending indicates what happens to Qi when it is being pushed down.)

Acupuncture Treatment

Acupuncture, whether done using traditional needles or by more modern techniques, such as electrostimulation or laser, requires extensive training. It should only be done by a qualified practitioner. You can, however, use acupressure and massage of acupuncture points, and there are complete instructions and explanations for you to follow (see chapter 7).

In the hands of a skilled practitioner, acupuncture is particularly effective for recovery from drug and alcohol dependency, for pain control, and for relief from depression, obsessive-compulsive disorders, phobias, and anxiety attacks. Acupuncture has been used for immune regulation and to treat allergies, gynecological disorders, infertility, and digestive tract disturbances, as well as to aid postoperative healing and to ease the side effects of Western cancer treatments.

Moxibustion

Moxibustion uses burning herbs, from the mugwort plant, placed on or near the body, to stimulate specific acupuncture points. This warms the Channels and expels Cold and Dampness, creates a smooth flow of Qi and Xue, strengthens Yang Qi, prevents disease, and maintains health.

For hundreds of years, moxibustion has been partnered with acupuncture or used alone as a modality. According to the Chinese text *Introduction to Medicine*, "When a disease fails to respond to medication and acupuncture, moxibustion is suggested."

There are many forms of moxibustion. A great modern book that describes all types of Chinese moxibustion treatment is *Moxibustion: A Modern Clinical Handbook* by Lorraine Wilcox. The two basic forms of moxibustion we use in my clinic are the cone and the stick. If directed by your practitioner, you can use both of them for self-care at home. Your practitioner can supply you with loose moxa or moxa sticks.

You make a moxa cone by compressing the herb mixture, known as moxa wool, into a cone about the size of the upper part of your thumb. The cone is then burned on the body. One of the most common applications is to the navel, where it is effective in relieving abdominal pain and diarrhea and in easing excessive sweating, cold limbs, and a flagging pulse. When moxa cones are burned on other parts of the body, the effect is to ease disharmonies in Channels and Organ Systems associated with those points.

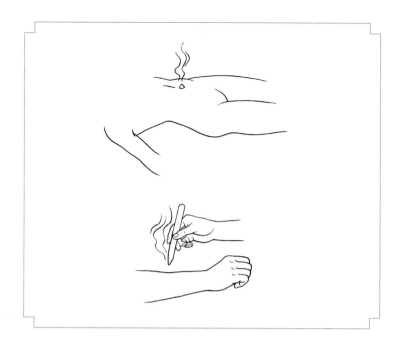

USING MOXA CONES

Before using moxa at home, discuss this treatment with your practitioner to make sure it is the correct treatment for you.

At home, never place the moxa cone directly on your skin!

1. Make three cones. Place each one firmly on a slice of dry aconite about ⅛ inch (2 mm) thick and set it within arm's reach. Aconite is a special herb your practitioner can give you or you can buy it from an herbalist. It may be toxic if ingested, but perfectly safe when used with the moxa cone. Instead of aconite, you may use a slice of fresh ginger about ⅛ inch (2 mm) thick that you have pierced with four or five small holes. *Note:* The ginger tends to spread the heat more than the aconite, and because it is damp, it doesn't offer as much insulation, so if you are using ginger, be especially careful not to burn your skin.

2. Lie down. Place a piece of clean cotton somewhere on your torso so you can retrieve it quickly if need be.

3. Put 2 tablespoons (30 g) of salt in your navel and tamp down until smooth and flat. (If you have an "outie," the Chinese texts suggest taking a long, wet noodle and forming a circle around the navel to contain the salt.)

4. Pick up the aconite (or ginger) with the cone on top. Light the cone—from the top if you want it to burn cooler and more slowly; from the bottom (don't light the aconite or ginger) if you want it to burn hotter and more rapidly. In my clinic, we light both the top and the bottom for even warmth. Place the aconite (or ginger) with the moxa on top of it over the salt.

5. If, as the moxa burns, it becomes too hot, gently lift the moxa and aconite (or ginger), slip the piece of cotton cloth over the salt, and set the aconite (or ginger) and moxa back in place.

6. Let the moxa burn down. If it still feels too hot, remove the aconite (or ginger) and cotton. Let the salt cool. Repeat three times. When you're done, save the aconite; brush off the salt. Throw away the ginger and cotton.

7. To place moxa cones on other points, skip the salt and use a piece of cotton topped with a slice of ginger or aconite.

USING MOXA STICKS

Moxa sticks, which are the size of big cigars, are available pre-rolled from your practitioner or an herbalist. When lit, they are used like wands by circling their burning ends over

"When a disease fails to respond to medication and acupuncture, moxibustion is suggested."

—Introduction to Medicine

various acupuncture points. This method is particularly effective in treating painful joints and chronic problems, such as painful periods, hernias, and abdominal pain.

To use a moxa stick, mark the acupuncture points you want to heat with a small dot. Light the stick with a match and let it burn until it begins to smoke. Holding it in the middle, bring the burning tip 1 inch (2.5 cm) from the skin. Hold your other hand next to the skin so you can feel if it gets too hot. (This is especially important if you are performing moxa on a partner.) Move it slowly in a clockwise circle over the point. If it feels too hot or the skin becomes too red, pull back in ½-inch (1.3 cm) intervals until it feels warming but not burning. Repeat until the area feels bathed in warmth, you can sense the Qi flowing from that spot, and you feel relaxed.

WARNING

To extinguish moxa sticks, don't use water or try to smash out the fire because if you do, they burn down and can't be reused. The best method is to cut off the supply of oxygen by wrapping the moxa in a piece of aluminum foil or placing it in a small glass container or bottle and completely closing the top. You can also ask your practitioner for a moxa snuffer, which is a special tool we use in the clinic to hold moxa sticks.

WHEN TO AVOID MOXIBUSTION

Moxa is contraindicated for Heat and Excess disharmonies or when there is a fever. Furthermore, at home pregnant women should avoid moxa on the abdominal and lumbo-sacral areas, although practitioners may use moxa in a clinic during pregnancy. Those with numbness in their arms, legs, feet, or toes or who suffer from narcolepsy should not do moxa on themselves. No one should do moxa in bed.

Moxa is performed over acupuncture points or areas of the body that need warmth or tonification. The following acupuncture points can be used for moxibustion treatment.

Ren 6: Located three fingers below the navel, tonifies Deficiency, tonifies Qi, strengthens the Kidney, and is good for gynecological disorders.

Ren 8: Located in the navel, tonifies Yang, warms the abdomen, strengthens Qi, and is good for all types of diarrhea and Coldness.

Stomach 36: Located four fingers below the knee, near the bone on the outer side of the leg. This is a major Qi point on the body, and it tonifies and regulates Qi, harmonizes the Stomach and the Spleen, and is good for digestive disorders and lack of energy.

Spleen 6: Located four fingers above the bone that sticks out of the inner ankle, known as the Three Yin Meeting Point, it tonifies the Spleen, Kidney, and Liver and is good for gynecologic and digestive disorders.

Ren 12: Located halfway between the navel and the tip of the sternum, effective in dispelling Dampness and treating digestive problems associated with Cold.

CHAPTER 6

EXERCISE AND MEDITATION

Exercise/meditation is the fourth pillar of Chinese medicine therapy. Without its Qi-balancing effects and benefits to mind/body/ spirit, wholeness cannot be achieved.

I recommend Qi Gong exercise and meditation to many of my clients as part of a total program. Qi Gong can be very important to the process of restoring harmony. For people who are not particularly interested in exercising, it offers you immediate gratification without having to go through a painful aerobics routine, joining an overcrowded health club, or spending money on equipment. If you are an exercise enthusiast, Qi Gong offers you many of the health benefits of running or weight training—without the risks.

Following is an introduction to several of the basic techniques, in hopes that you will integrate them into your exercise routines, expanding your definition of physical fitness and experimenting with ways of combining Eastern exercise with Western sports activities. Your expert guide is Larry Wong, an accomplished practitioner and teacher.

Qi Gong 101: Understanding the Chinese Concept of Exercise/Meditation

by Larry Wong

Welcome. I am Larry Wong, and I am going to introduce you to what I know of the art of Qi Gong. I urge you to keep in mind that there are many approaches to Qi Gong. Each one provides far-reaching health benefits. With Qi Gong, you may learn the principles and gain the benefits from any number of approaches.

Qi Gong, which combines meditative and physically active elements, is the basic exercise system within Chinese medicine. Qi Gong practice is designed to help you preserve your Jing, strengthen and balance the flow of Qi, and enlighten your Shen. Its dynamic exercises and meditations have Yin and Yang aspects: The Yin is *being* it; the Yang is *doing* it. Yin exercises are expressed through relaxed stretching, visualization, and breathing. Yang exercises are expressed in a more aerobic or dynamic way. They are particularly effective for supporting the immune system. In China, Qi Gong is used extensively for people with cancer.

Anyone of any age or physical condition can do Qi Gong. You don't have to be able to run a marathon or bench press a car to pursue healthfulness and enjoy the benefits. When you design your exercise/meditation practice, you will pick what suits your individual constitution. Some of us are born with one type of constitution; some with another. We each have inherited imbalances that we cannot control but with which we must work. That's why for some people it is easier to achieve balance and strength than it is for others. But whatever your nature, Qi Gong can help you become the most balanced you can be.

Qi Gong is truly a system for a lifetime. That's why so many people over age sixty in China practice Qi Gong and Tai Chi. The effects may be powerful, but the routines themselves are usually gentle. Even the dynamic exercises—some of which explode the Qi—use forcefulness in different ways than in the West. The following are some effects of Qi Gong.

Maintaining health: Qi Gong helps maintain health by creating a state of mental and physical calmness, which indicates that Qi is balanced and harmonious. This allows the mind/body/spirit to function most efficiently, with the least amount of stress.

When you start practicing Qi Gong, the primary goal is to concentrate on letting go. That's because most imbalance comes from holding on to too much for too long. Most of us are familiar with physical strength of muscles, and when we think about exercising, we think in terms of tensing muscles. Qi is different. Qi strength is revealed by a smooth, calm, concentrated effort that is free of stress and does not pit one part of the body against another.

Managing illness: It's harder to remedy an illness than to prevent it, and Qi Gong has powerful preventive effects. However, when disharmony becomes apparent, Qi Gong also can play a crucial role in restoring harmony.

Qi Gong movement and postures are shaped by the principle of Yin/Yang: the complementary interrelationship of qualities such as fast and slow, hard and soft, Excess or Deficiency, and External and Internal. Qi Gong uses these contrasting and complementary qualities to restore harmony to the Essential Substances, Organ Systems, and Channels.

Waging combat: Around 500 CE, in the Liang Dynasty, Qi Gong was adopted by various martial artists to increase stamina and power. For the most part, the breathing, concentration, and agility were assets to the warriors and improved their well-being.

Attaining enlightenment: Buddhist monks who use Qi Gong in their pursuit for higher consciousness and enlightenment concentrate on Qi Gong's ability to influence their Shen. Mastering Marrow Washing allows the practitioner to gain so much control over the flow of Qi that he or she can direct it into the forehead and elevate consciousness. The rest of us can enjoy the influence of Qi Gong on our Shen, but at a lower level.

Whatever reason you use Qi Gong, the practice should raise your Qi to a higher state if you increase concentration, practice controlled breathing, and execute the Qi Gong routines.

THE BASIC TECHNIQUES

Here are the basic Qi Gong techniques.

Concentration: Concentration leads to and results from Qi awareness, breathing techniques, and Qi Gong exercises. It is a process of focusing in and letting go at the same time. Through deep relaxation and expanding your consciousness, you are able to create a frame of mind that is large enough to encompass your entire mind/body/spirit's functions, yet focused enough to allow outside distractions, worries, and everyday hassles to drift away.

This inward focus that expands outward to join you with the rhythms of the universe epitomizes Yin/Yang. Yin tends to be more expansive, and Yang more concentrated. You discover your Yin/Yang balance by treating Yin and Yang as ingredients in a recipe: Add a bit more Yin, toss in a dash of Yang to make the mixture suit your constitution or circumstances. Some people need more or less Yin or Yang, depending upon the situation.

You will find that as you do exercise/meditation you become more adept at this form of concentration, because it is the natural expression of the practice. As you learn to concentrate more effectively, you will find you have greater power to affect Qi through the various Qi Gong exercises in this chapter or through the use of other focused meditations and Tai Chi.

Breathing: In the sixth century BCE, Lao Tzu first described breathing techniques as a way to stimulate Qi. From there, two types of breathing evolved: Buddha's Breath and Taoist's Breath. Both methods infuse the body with Qi and help focus meditation.

- **Buddha's Breath:** When you inhale, extend your abdomen, filling it with air. When you exhale, contract your abdomen, expelling the air from the bottom of your lungs first and then pushing it up and out until your abdomen and chest are deflated. You may want to practice inhaling for a slow count of eight and exhaling for a count of sixteen. As you breathe in and out, imagine inviting your Qi to flow through the Channels. Use your mind to invite the Qi to flow; you want to guide the flow, not tug at it or push it.

- **Taoist's Breath:** The pattern is the opposite of above. When you breathe in, you contract your abdominal muscles. When you exhale, you relax the torso and lungs.

QI GONG ROUTINES

There are two basic types of Qi Gong activities: Wei Dan (external elixir) and Nei Dan (internal elixir). Both focus on strengthening and balancing the Qi by using dynamic routines and still postures, but they approach the tasks in two different ways.

Wei Dan

This practice focuses exercises on the muscles to build up your Qi until it becomes so concentrated that it overflows and runs out from where it has collected, through the Channels, and into all parts of your body.

In dynamic, moving Wei Dan exercises, muscles are tensed and released over and over again with complete concentration. The tension should be as light as possible because tension causes Stagnant Qi, which is the very antithesis of what you want to accomplish. In fact, it is often suggested that you simply *imagine* that you are tensing the muscles. After several minutes, the generated Qi warms the muscles.

Typical routines that use dynamic, moving Wei Dan exercises include the Dan Mo or Muscle/Tendon Changing Classic. In this routine, you slightly tense or imagine you are tensing isolated limb muscles, such as your forearm, your palm, your wrist, your biceps, and your shoulder, and then relax completely. Concentration and breath control are vital components of the process.

There are other moving Wei Dan routines that call for moving your legs, torso, and arms into specific positions to relax or massage the Organ Systems. For example, you may extend and stretch your arms over your head, then hold and relax, thus massaging the Lung Channel and Lung Organ System more enthusiastically than with the less mobile Dan Mo style.

In the still Wei Dan exercises, muscle groups are targeted but not tensed. For example, hold your arms fully extended, palms down, out to the sides of your body. Don't tighten muscles, but hold that position for at least a minute—building up to longer—until the arms begin to shake or feel warm. When you let your arms fall to your sides and relax, shrugging your shoulder muscles and shaking your hands gently, the accumulated Qi is sent coursing out through the Channels. In this manner, Qi is stimulated at various locations in the body by continual muscular exertion combined with concentration.

Wei Dan practice is relatively simple to learn, and it provides immediate benefits. But it is not a lesser form of Qi Gong. Even masters of the more arcane processes use Wei Dan for its Qi strengthening powers.

Nei Dan

This is a more demanding, less easy to master, and more time-consuming form of Qi Gong. It uses mental powers to

"Breathing can direct Qi through the body like the wind filling the sails of a ship."

direct Qi through the Channels. You must have a teacher to guide you and to help you avoid the potential risks associated with doing the practice incorrectly.

In one Nei Dan exercise, you concentrate Qi on the Dantien (below the navel) and then disperse it through the body using the powers of the mind. Qi may travel in the following three pathways:

- **The Fire Path:** In the Fire Path, you build Qi in the abdomen through breathing and/or thought, and once it accumulates sufficiently, you direct it with your mind along the two Extraordinary Channels known as the Conception Channel and the Governing Channel. This is known as the Small Circulation. The next level is to move Qi through the remaining six Extraordinary Channels. This is called the Grand Circulation.

- **The Wind Path:** In the Wind Path, Qi moves in the opposite direction as it did on the Fire Path.

- **The Water Path:** In the Water Path, Qi moves through the spine and is used in Marrow Washing to prolong life and increase enlightenment.

BREATHING EXERCISES

Breathing can direct Qi through the body like the wind filling the sails of a ship. Breathing exercises can invigorate or sedate, depending on how you use them.

On alternate days, practice the following routine, using Buddha's Breath and Taoist's Breath breathing techniques. (See both "Buddha's Breath" and "Taoist's Breath" on page 132.)

Sit on the floor with your legs crossed in lotus or cross-legged style. This is important so that Qi does not enter and become Stagnant in the lower body, but follows the breathing path through your torso and your head.

Inhale to a count of four to eight, depending on what you are comfortable with. For Buddha's Breath, extend your belly, filling it up from the bottom. For Taoist's Breath, inhale, contracting your abdomen, and exhale, letting your abdomen relax outward.

As you inhale, turn your attention to your nose. Guide the Qi downward from your nose toward the Dantien, 1 to 2 inches (2.5 to 5 cm) below the navel. Women should not concentrate on the Dantien during their periods. Concentrate on your solar plexus instead.

Exhale to a count of eight to sixteen and move the Qi down the torso, around your pelvic region, and up to your tailbone.

Inhale and move the Qi up the back to the top of your shoulders.

Exhale and move the Qi up the back of your head and back to your nose.

If you cannot feel the Qi clearly, patience and practice will make it more apparent. Once you are comfortable with this practice, you may increase the pace by completing the cycle in one inhalation and one exhalation. On the inhalation, move Qi from your nose to your tailbone. On the exhalation, move Qi from your tailbone back to your nose.

Thanks again to Sifu Larry Wong for his generosity in sharing his insight, expertise, and practice of Qi Gong.

Meditation

In this section are meditations that we recommend at Chicken Soup Chinese Medicine.

As a beginner, you want to allow yourself the time and pleasure of learning to meditate. If it feels awkward or if you have difficulty maintaining concentration, take a step back.

Don't set your standards too high. If you expect too much too soon, you disturb your mind/body/spirit and promote restlessness, frustration, and stress. This may defeat the whole purpose of meditation.

DON'T FEEL THE BURN

Many people come into my clinic suffering from the fanatic pursuit of Western exercise: sore muscles, bruised bones, twisted ankles, sore backs, tension, and stress. These frequent injuries occur in part because the concept of exercise has become distorted. Feel the burn. Bop 'til you drop. No pain, no gain. This notion of exercise often injures the mind/body/spirit; it makes us sore and exhausted instead of agile and refreshed. For some people, it damages the Qi by reducing energy. They end up feeling generally fatigued overall. For other people, exercise has become a kind of poison to the system instead of an expression of the joyous unity of mind/body/spirit.

In contrast, Qi Gong exercise/meditation is a unified process dedicated to creating balance, strength, agility, and grace that assures vitality through old age.

Your first goal should be simply to be quiet, relaxed, and comfortable for a few minutes.

Try to meditate in a comfortable environment. As you progress, distractions will become less of a problem. In the beginning, you want to eliminate as many distractions as possible. Choose a quiet room that is not so warm that you fall asleep nor so cold that you tense up. Wear loose-fitting clothing. Turn on meditation music to help block outside noise if need be.

Find a posture that works for you. Not everyone can sit on the floor in a full or half lotus or cross-legged. You may want to lie down, sit in a straight-backed chair, or stand.

Don't eat heavy foods or drink alcohol or caffeine before meditating.

Don't hold on to disturbing thoughts. One of the goals of meditation is to disconnect from worries. If you've had a tough day at work, a disagreement with your spouse, or worries about money, each exhalation of breath is a chance to let a piece of that tension dissipate.

QI MEDITATION

The following is a meditation/visualization that is designed to help you tune in to the motion of Qi throughout the Channels and to help in the body's natural process of self-healing. The first few times you do this meditation, you can have someone read it to you in a gentle, slow voice, cuing you as to the steps. You can also tape this in your own voice and listen to it as you go through the meditation. Eventually, you will be able to go through the steps silently.

Get into a comfortable position. Allow your body to begin to relax. Close your eyes. Close your mouth and place the tip of your tongue against the roof of your mouth. This connects the Yin and Yang Channels and allows for Qi flow.

With your eyes closed, bring your attention to the area around and below your navel; in Japanese it is called the *hara*; in Chinese it's called the *Dantien.* This is one area where Qi is stored.

Allow yourself to begin to breathe into the area. You may use either breathing technique.

As you breathe into your abdomen, into your belly, into the Dantien, notice a warmth from the center of your abdomen, beginning as a small glow and getting brighter and brighter until there is a ball of light filling your abdomen. Allow yourself to feel this ball of light, any color that you'd like.

Now, as you breathe, notice the energy moving up into the area of your heart and opening up into your chest.

Next, feel it move to the area in front of your arm, just below the shoulder bone. This energy moves from the area below your shoulder bone, down the outside of your arm all the way to your thumb, on the inside of your thumb. Feel the warmth and the movement of energy down the Lung Channel.

When it gets to the end of the Lung Channel at the tip of the thumb, move your focus over to your index finger, where the Large Intestine Channel begins.

The Qi then moves through your hand, up the outside of the arm, coming up over your shoulder, up the side of your neck, and up to the outside of your nose. Then move to the Stomach Channel that begins below your eye. It flows down the neck, over the front of your body, through your chest, down outside your navel, around your pubic area, then down the outside of your leg, to a very important point, just below

"Let go of disturbing thoughts."

your knee, where the energy of the body becomes very strong. It then moves on down across the front of your foot and into the top of your toes, where it meets the Spleen Channel.

The Spleen Channel allows food energy to move through the body and impacts digestion.

Begin inside your big toe, coming up the arch of your foot, in front of your ankle bone, on the inside of your leg, all the way up by your knee, continuing inside your leg, and up the front of your body, curving around your ribs, and ending in your costal (rib) area.

The Spleen Channel then connects internally with the Heart Channel.

The Heart Channel emerges from your heart into the centers of your armpits, moving down the insides of your arms, all the way to your small fingers, where it attaches to the Small Intestine Channel.

The Small Intestine Channel is a very good Channel to help open up the brain.

This Channel runs up the outside of the arms, coming all the way back up, across your scapulas, up the back of your neck, and around your ears, where it ends in front of your ears.

This connects to the Urinary Bladder Channel, the longest Channel, at the insides of your eyes.

From your eyes, the Channel comes up across the top of your head and down the back of your neck, where it splits into two parallel lines, which then extend down your whole back on either side of your spine, connecting the organs together.

The two rows of the Urinary Bladder Channel are side by side, and they connect again at the back of your buttocks, coming down the backs of the middles of your legs through your knees, all the way down your legs, around your ankle bones, and into your little toes.

The Urinary Bladder Channel connects with the Kidney Channel on the very bottom of your feet. The Kidney Channel moves up from your feet, around the insides of your ankles, all the way up the insides of your legs, and up around your navel. And this Channel comes all the way up to the upper part of your chest, where there are some of the most important points in Chinese medicine for meditation and connection with the Shen.

Here the Kidney Channel connects with the Pericardium Channel, which starts in front of your arms, moves down the very middle of your arms, into the palms of your hands, and to your middle fingers, where it then connects with the Triple Burner Channel, the Channel that helps regulate the temperature of your body. The Triple Burner Channel begins on your fourth fingers, comes up over the top of your hands, all the way up your arms and around your elbows, over your shoulders, and up your neck and around your ears, where it connects with the Gallbladder Channel.

The Gallbladder Channel is the most crooked Channel on the body. It zigzags across the top of your head, comes down the back of your neck, across your shoulders, and down the sides of your body, zigzagging again on the sides of your body, and all the way down over your hips and the deepest point in the muscle of your body in your buttocks, then moves down the side of your legs, all the way down to the top of your toes, to the fourth toes.

You pick up the Liver Channel on the big toes. It comes across the top of your feet, and again toward the insides of your feet and around your ankles, up the middle of the inside of your legs by your knees, and all the way up the inside of your legs. This Channel circles the genital area, coming up into your rib cage near the Liver, yet on both sides of your body. And then we return again to the Lung Channel.

Once you have completed the cycle, sit or lie peacefully, allowing yourself time to make your transition back to your surrounding environment in a graceful manner.

LOTUS BLOSSOM MEDITATION

This is one of my favorite meditations. It is a brief and simple meditation that can be done almost anywhere, any time you feel the need to ease stress or allow your feelings of affection and connection to expand.

Sit peacefully, breathing evenly.

Half close your eyes.

Inhale slowly, filling your body with air.

At the same time, concentrate your attention on the area of the fourth chakra that is located at your breastbone in the center of your chest.

Imagine a beautiful lotus blossom. Its petals are closed, and its scent is but a promise.

As you exhale, see that blossom unfold. The velvety smooth petals extend, reaching out, releasing a beautiful scent.

Inhale and smell the fragrant aroma.

The petals are opening ever further. And as they open, you feel your heart and chest opening up to the world, expanding, relaxing.

You may extend the opening petals as far as you want. Feel your heart open in the same proportion.

When you have arrived at an openness that is comfortable, hold it there as you enjoy the scent of the flower and breathe in and out slowly.

You may practice this meditation concentrating on a chakra, or energy center. Particularly effective are the third chakra, located at the diaphragm, and the second chakra, located below the navel in the Dantien or hara area.

CHAPTER 7

MASSAGE AND OTHER FORMS OF BODY THERAPY

Massage, whether done solo, with a partner, or by a professional massage therapist, offers the energy of acupuncture, the serenity of meditation, and the spiritual refreshment that comes through being touched. Massage is an important part of your everyday health care routine. Just as you strive to integrate the dietary guidelines from chapter 3 and the exercise/meditation guidelines from chapter 6 into your daily self-care habits, so should you make room for massage as part of the routine you follow to strengthen your immune system and maintain your balance.

In this chapter, we look at Chinese Qi Gong self-massage, self-acupressure, and self-ear acupressure. There are many other forms of massage—such as Shiatsu, Western Reflexology, deep tissue, lymphatic drainage, and Swedish—each valuable for restoring harmony. Although these forms of massage are not presented in detail in this book, you may want to explore them. They can be integrated into your comprehensive programs for preventive care and/or to treat disharmony.

Qi Gong Massage

Qi Gong massage is an extension of Qi Gong exercise/ meditation. Among the more skilled masters of the art, self-massage can be done with the mind, moving Qi and Xue through the Channels, relaxing muscles, and massaging Organ Systems mentally. For the rest of us, manual Qi Gong massage—done on ourselves or with a partner or practitioner—is an important part of any preventive health care program, because regular massage helps nourish the mind/body/spirit and maintains harmony in all systems.

WARNING

It is best if you do not perform self-massage or have a massage done to you on any area where you have a skin eruption, a localized infection, swelling, or localized malignancies, or where you've had very recent surgery. Pregnant women should have massage on the abdomen and torso only from a professional massage therapist.

If you exercise three or more times a week, go through the complete Ten-Step Qi-Xue Self-Massage once a week. Use the specific self-massage routines for hand, ear, head, or foot as you feel the need.

If you are sedentary, have an injury that's preventing you from exercising, or simply find you're stuck at a desk and cannot exercise for a given period of time, do the foot and head massage every other day and practice the Ten-Step Qi-Xue Self-Massage once or twice a week. You will help prevent the formation of disharmonies in the flow of Essential Substances and consequent problems in the Organ Systems.

The benefits of Qi Gong massage include working on the Channels to improve circulation of Essential Substances, particularly Qi and Xue; dilation of the blood vessels; stimulation of the lymph system and elimination of wastes and toxins; improved muscle tone; relief of stress and promotion of relaxation and sleep—and it just makes you feel good.

TEN-STEP QI-XUE SELF-MASSAGE

Based on the flow of the Essential Substances through the Channels and Organ Systems, this massage series provides you with a complete relaxation and rejuvenation routine. You may use all or any part of it any time you feel the need for a little repair work and a bit of TLC.

Establish a slow, rhythmic pattern of breathing while doing self-massage. Inhale slowly for the count of three and exhale slowly for the count of six. As you become more comfortable with this entire series of exercises, try to inhale every time you change the position of your hands and exhale while you massage yourself. The count will give you an even tempo.

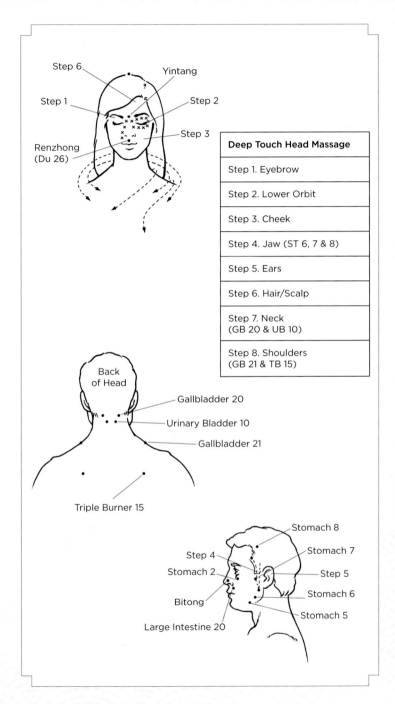

Deep Touch Head Massage
Step 1. Eyebrow
Step 2. Lower Orbit
Step 3. Cheek
Step 4. Jaw (ST 6, 7 & 8)
Step 5. Ears
Step 6. Hair/Scalp
Step 7. Neck (GB 20 & UB 10)
Step 8. Shoulders (GB 21 & TB 15)

Step 6
Yintang
Step 1
Step 2
Step 3
Renzhong (Du 26)

Back of Head
Gallbladder 20
Urinary Bladder 10
Gallbladder 21
Triple Burner 15

Stomach 8
Stomach 7
Step 4
Step 5
Stomach 2
Stomach 6
Bitong
Stomach 5
Large Intestine 20

Step One: General Head Massage

Massage promotes general relaxation and the harmonious flow of Qi and Xue. It is particularly good if you are suffering from chronic sinusitis, respiratory allergies, temporomandibular joint disorder (TMJ), headaches, and anxiety or depression.

Using your middle fingers, massage the bridge of your nose on both sides. Complete five circular rubbing motions, moving from the top to the outside, down toward your nose, and then into the point above the inside corner of your eye.

Move your hands up from the bridge to the top center of your forehead.

Spread your hands apart, with the fingers of your right hand moving down to the right temple and fingers of the left hand moving down to the left temple. Massage the temple in a circular motion five times.

Move your hands up to the top of your head and bring them down to your neck. Rub the back of your neck up and down, along the tendons that extend on either side, five times.

Move your hands to the outside of the neck until you can feel the lower point of your jaw joint.

Rub that five times.

Now move your hands back to the bridge of your nose and in a smooth motion trace the outline of your eyebrows to your temple and then move your hand down to the hollow of your cheek.

Repeat this motion three times.

Slowly rotate your head around, stretching your neck so your right ear is almost touching your right shoulder. Then slowly shift your head to the front so your chin is touching your chest. Then swing your head to the left so the left ear is almost touching the left shoulder. Now move it slowly toward the back. Look up at the ceiling. Repeat three times, then reverse direction and repeat again.

Step Two: Eye Massage

To improve the circulation of Qi and Xue and improve visual clarity, you want to direct Qi to your eyes.

Place your index and middle fingers on the inside points of your eyebrows. Massage in a circular motion five times.

Move your fingers to the outer corner of your eyes and rub gently.

Move your fingers down from the corners of your eyes to the top of your jawbone. Then move the fingers slowly down the length of your lower jaw until they almost meet at your chin.

Place your palms together and rub them back and forth across each other until they become quite warm. Cup your hands over your eyes to share your hand Qi with them. Do not touch your eyes.

Step Three: General Ear Massage

Use of general ear massage tonifies the whole body—every Organ System, the joints, and all body parts—and keeps your hearing healthy.

If you are wearing large earrings, take them off. Using your two middle fingers, gently rub around the entire ear several times.

Place your thumbs inside your ears and your fingers along the widest part of the ear flap. Now pull gently outward so the thumb moves from the inside to the outer edge of the ear. Hold for a count of three. Repeat three times.

Take each ear lobe between your thumbs and forefingers and rub gently, pulling downward.

Place your palms over your ears and massage the entire ear. Repeat five times.

Press your palms against your ears and then remove quickly.

Shake out your hands and fingers. Sit quietly for two minutes.

Step Four: Neck Massage

This moves Qi and Xue along the spine.

Sit with your back straight and your head tipped ever so slightly forward.

Place your hands together in a prayer position. Open your fingers and then curl your fingers, allowing them to interweave. Spread your palms apart so your fingers are lying across the backs of your hands and both palms are parallel to the floor.

Place your hands like a cradle against the back of your skull. Your thumbs should be pointing straight down on either side of your neck.

Massage the tendons beneath your thumbs from top to bottom. Repeat five times.

Raise your thumbs up slightly to catch the point at the base of your skull where the bone meets the neck. Rub back and forth along this ridge. Go very slowly, probing the area, feeling where you want to apply more or less pressure. When you find the spot that is particularly tender to the touch, hold your thumb there for a slow count of six. Exhale while holding the point. Repeat as many times as you like.

Step Five: Torso Massage

This step and the following one are important for anyone who wants to keep the Lung System clear and the Heart

Xue flowing smoothly. The steps are particularly helpful for digestive problems, asthma symptoms, and congestion.

Open your palms. Place them on the front of your neck. Moving your hands from your neck to the front of your body, glide over your chest with long smooth strokes of your open palms.

Repeat several times.

Cross your arms. Using your first and second fingers, massage a point about 2 inches (5 cm) above the center of each nipple. Circle your fingers on the right hand over your left nipple, then your left hand over your right nipple. You may feel your lungs open up.

Placing your palms flat on each side of your torso (left hand on left side, right hand on right side), move the Qi (from the point above your nipple that you just massaged) to the side and bottom of your lungs. Massage in a smooth flat motion to the side of your torso and then down to your diaphragm.

Step Six: Qi Up, Qi Down

Place the tips of the fingers of your right hand on the pectoral muscle by the crook of your left arm.

Move your fingers in a circular motion, tracing a 3-inch (7.5 cm) circle from the top of your chest moving inward, down, to the outside and back up to the top. Repeat this, creating a spiral shape vertically down a line through the nipple. As you go in this direction (only!) move your hand down the full length of your torso.

Repeat the massage using the tips of your left-hand fingers on the right side of the torso. Make sure that you move your fingers from the top of your torso, toward your breastbone, then to your toes, and finally toward your arm.

Step Seven: Abdominal Massage

This technique is helpful for anyone with digestive problems, PMS, or cramps, and it helps harmonize the Large Intestine, Small Intestine, Liver, Spleen, Stomach, and Gallbladder. You may want to use oil infused with cinnamon to warm your belly if it is generally Cold during your period or if you have loose stools and abdominal cramps due to Cold.

Lie on a flat, firm surface. If needed, place a small pillow under your knees to take strain off your lower back.

So there is less distraction, close your eyes halfway. Inhale slowly and deeply.

Place your right palm on your stomach, above your navel, with your thumb lying against the skin pointing toward your chin. Place your left hand so it is on top of the right. Breath in and out slowly, feeling the warmth under your hands. (If you are left-handed, place your left hand on your stomach first.)

Rub your stomach gently in a clockwise motion. Repeat twenty to forty times.

Raise your hands up to the lower edge of your rib cage on either side of your torso. Smoothly massage down the length of your lower torso into the pelvic area and the groin. Repeat five times.

Now move your hand to the center of your abdomen below your navel. Repeat the motion as above.

Sit facing forward; inhale. Turn your head and neck, but not your torso, and look over your left shoulder. Exhale. Now inhale as you turn your head and neck and look over your right shoulder. Exhale.

Take your right hand and place it along your waist on the left side of your body. Inhale. As you exhale slowly, move your palm forward along your waistline toward your navel. Reverse.

With your palm open and flat, rub the front of your lower torso over your hip bones and down onto the tops of your thighs. Use one long, slow motion.

Return to the first position with your right hand over your stomach and your left hand on top of the right. Slowly, gently, rub in a clockwise motion for the count of six. Breathe in on the count of three and out on the count of six. Keep your eyelids at half-mast.

Step Eight: Circulating the Lower Qi and Xue

To promote harmonious flow of Qi and Xue, a complete massage keeps the motion going from your head through your feet in a complete cycle. If you are going to complete the massage cycle, remain seated with your feet flat on the floor about 8 inches (20 cm) apart.

Sit on a firm, un-upholstered, but comfortable chair without arms. Sit with good posture, but not stiffly. Rub your inner thighs with the same circular motion that you applied to your torso, always moving in a circle that goes from the top of the thigh (twelve o'clock), down the outside toward nine o'clock, and up through six and three o'clock. Spiral down your thighs to your knees. Repeat three times.

Using your thumbs, press gently but firmly on the top center of your thighs and draw your thumbs down to your knees. If you feel any tender spots, stop at that point and gently vibrate your thumb back and forth. Repeat three times.

When you come down to the top of your knees for the last time, hold your thumbs in place and put your fingers across the center of the kneecaps. Rub gently. Then rub your hands down the outside of your calves, from top to bottom (but not back up) five times.

Cross one leg over the other so your calf is in easy reach and lying parallel with the floor.

Place your fingers in the ridge that is formed between the near side of your shin bone and the calf muscle. Slowly move your fingers down from your knee to your ankle. Press with a firm, steady motion. If any point is tender, move your fingers in a circular motion on the point. Go from the top to the bottom. Repeat as desired with your other leg.

Step Nine: General Foot Massage

In Chinese medicine, the feet play a crucial role in the functioning of the Channels. They are also associated with the harmonious balance of the Organ Systems and Essential Substances.

To help promote smooth flow of Qi and Xue and keep the Channels working smoothly, you can give yourself a general foot massage, rubbing each part of the foot, starting with your ankle and ending with your toes. Devote extra effort to rubbing your toes and pay attention to the areas between your toes and between the long, thin bones that run along the top of your foot. Foot massage oil can provide an extra soothing touch. Use peppermint-infused oil if you are Hot, and use cinnamon-infused oil if you are Cold.

As you rub your feet, you may want to target several acupuncture points for acupressure. Particularly important points to rub include:

Kidney 1, directly in the center of each foot right below the ball, is an important point to help keep the Kidney System working harmoniously, which impacts the functioning of all the other Organ Systems.

Spleen 4, Liver 3, and Gallbladder 41 are also important foot points to help harmonize Qi and the Organ Systems.

Step Ten: Arm and Hand Massage

After your arms and hands have worked hard massaging the rest of your body, it's their turn to be pampered.

An arm massage should be done from your shoulder to the tips of your fingers in long, slow strokes along the inside and the outside of your biceps and forearm. Rub between or along the bones, rather than on top of them.

After you extend the Qi through your arm, return to the acupuncture point, Large Intestine 14, at the outside of the biceps below the armpit, the crook of the elbow, and the

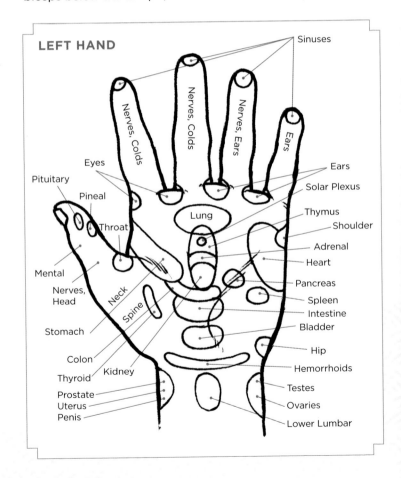

LEFT HAND

Sinuses

Nerves, Colds

Nerves, Colds

Nerves, Ears

Ears

Eyes

Ears

Pituitary

Solar Plexus

Pineal

Thymus

Throat

Lung

Shoulder

Adrenal

Heart

Mental

Pancreas

Nerves, Head

Neck

Spine

Spleen

Intestine

Bladder

Stomach

Hip

Colon

Hemorrhoids

Kidney

Thyroid

Testes

Prostate

Ovaries

Uterus

Penis

Lower Lumbar

back of the wrist. On these points, press slowly and evenly. Breathe deeply.

A general hand massage can be done with your thumb moving in a gentle clockwise motion from your wrist to your fingertips, concentrating on the tissue between the bones and the areas around the knuckles and fingertips.

Once you've covered the entire surface of the hand, pull each finger out gently and rub the last section of your finger at the tip. Shake out your hands.

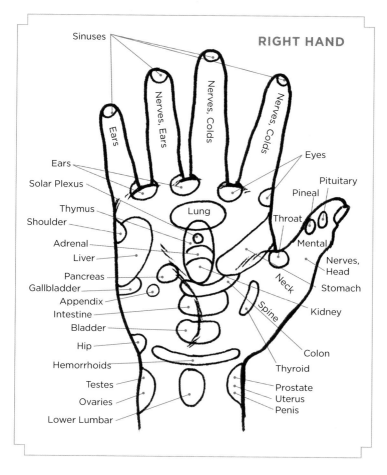

Sinuses

RIGHT HAND

Nerves, Ears

Nerves, Colds

Nerves, Colds

Ears

Nerves, Ears

Eyes

Ears

Pituitary

Solar Plexus

Pineal

Thymus

Lung

Shoulder

Throat

Adrenal

Mental

Liver

Nerves, Head

Pancreas

Neck

Stomach

Gallbladder

Spine

Appendix

Kidney

Intestine

Bladder

Hip

Colon

Hemorrhoids

Thyroid

Testes

Prostate

Ovaries

Uterus

Penis

Lower Lumbar

Acupressure Massage

Acupressure massage uses the thumb and hands to stimulate the acupuncture points along the Channels. If you are massaging someone else, to gain maximum effect without hurting yourself or straining your hand, use the following guidelines:

- Work the points with the soft, padded part of your thumb—where your thumbprint is.

- Press down firmly and smoothly.

- Don't jab or stab at a point.

- Always brace your thumb with the rest of your hand and fingers. For example, if you are massaging a point on your thigh, place your hand flat along the skin. Move your thumb into position, leaving the rest of your hand in contact with your leg. Press with your thumb. For more pressure or better leverage, don't pick up your hand. If you are massaging someone else, raise yourself up over her or him and press downward. If you are massaging yourself, lean into the pressure.

FOR ALERTNESS

Stomach 36 is located four finger widths from the hollow made when the knee is bent (below the kneecap) on the outside of the leg and one finger width over from the crest of the shin bone. Stimulating this point is also good for digestive problems, boosts energy, and is said by the Chinese to help strengthen the immune system. Stomach 36 was known in the old days as *Three Miles*, because when people hiked or walked to the point of exhaustion, if they stopped and rubbed that point, they were able to go 3 miles (4.8 km) more.

WARNING

Do not stimulate Large Intestine 4 when pregnant.

Large Intestine 4 is located in the webbing between the thumb and index finger. Press into the hollow against the bone from the index finger that extends down the length of the back of the hand. This point is also good for any problems above the neck, such as sinus problems and headaches. It is also beneficial for general inflammation, constipation, and diarrhea.

Stomach 36 is located four finger widths from the hollow made when the knee is bent (below the kneecap) on the outside of the leg and one finger width over from the crest of the shin bone.

Large Intestine 4 is located between the thumb and forefinger in the middle of the forefinger bone that goes from the knuckle to the wrist.

Liver 3 is located at the point where the bones of the big toe and the second toe meet and form a V. The point is slightly in front of their junction.

Lung 7 is located 1½ inches (3.8 cm) above the transverse wrist crease on the back of the hand. It is above the large bump on the outside of the wrist bone.

Kidney 3 is located on the inside of the ankle in the depression between the tip of the ankle bone and the Achilles tendon.

WARNING

During pregnancy, acupressure and acupuncture should be received only from a practitioner skilled in management of pregnancy.

FOR LOW BACK PAIN

Kidney 3 is located on the inside of the ankle in the depression between the tip of the ankle bone and the Achilles tendon. This is also good for immune support.

Urinary Bladder 60 is located midway between the ankle bone on the outside of the leg and the Achilles tendon, opposite Kidney 3.

Urinary Bladder 40 can be found in the center of the back of the knee. Points across the back of the knee correspond to the lumbar (lower back) vertebrae, so massage the entire crease. It is also good to massage down from Urinary Bladder 40 to Urinary Bladder 60.

Du 26 is located one-third of the distance between the bottom of the nose and the center of the top lip, in the slight indentation. This is known as the emergency point, and it is used if someone loses consciousness. For acute back pain, stand up and hold on to the back of a chair with one hand. With the other, press relatively hard on the point with your fingernail while you move the back gently in and out of the area of pain by swaying your hips and torso.

Pericardium 7 is in the middle of the wrist crease on the inside of the arm. It is also good for irregular heartbeat and tachycardia.

FOR GENERAL PAIN

Pericardium 6 is located on the inside of the wrist three finger widths above the wrist crease, between the two bones. Also good for anxiety, nausea, and morning sickness.

Pericardium 6 with Triple Burner 5: Triple Burner 5 is located three finger widths above the wrist crease on the top of the arm between the two long arm bones. Press Triple Burner 5 and Pericardium 6 at the same time for extra relief. This is good for carpal tunnel problems. These points are regulating points, and they enhance overall calmness.

Ren 17 is located between the nipples at the center of the chest. It is used to release grief and improve breath by regulating Zong Qi. It is also the area that holds the Ancestral Qi.

Yintang is located between the eyebrows in the center of the bridge of your nose. It is used to ease pain and release tension. It is good for headaches and overall relaxation.

FOR THE SHOULDER

Triple Burner 4 is found on the top side of the wrist at the midpoint of the wrist crease, between the two arm bones.

Triple Burner 5 is located three finger widths above the wrist crease on the top of the arm between the two long arm bones.

Small Intestine 3 is located in the indentation below the little finger knuckle on the outside of the hand. It is good for the neck and shoulders. If you have a stiff neck, rotate your neck in and out of the area of stiffness while pressing the point. It is also good for clearing the mind.

FOR THE MID-BACK

Liver 3 is located at the point where the bones of the big toe and the second toe meet and form a V. The point is slightly in front of their junction.

Gallbladder 40 is in the hollow indentation just to the front of the outside ankle bone.

FOR GYNECOLOGICAL PROBLEMS

Spleen 6 is located four finger widths above the tip of the inside ankle bone behind the shin bone.

Ren 4 and 6: Divide the line that runs from the navel to the pubic bone into five equal sections. Ren 4 is three sections below the navel. Ren 6 is one and a half sections below the navel.

AMAZING EAR MASSAGE

If the eyes are the windows to the soul, then the ears are the road maps. Located in the external part of those two little organs are acupuncture points that provide a direct route to all of the important functions of the mind/body/spirit.

Ear acupuncture points can be as powerful—or even more so—than points located on the Channels. For example, the three "no smoking points," known as Shenmen, Sympathetic, and Lung, are extremely effective in promoting nicotine detoxification.

To rub ear points, you may use your finger or a cotton swab or you can purchase an ear massage probe online or at a natural health store. Don't worry about touching other points. You'll be able to tell when you're in the right position. Ear points become very sensitive and tender when there is a disharmony in the corresponding part of the body.

Ear Acupuncture Points

Toe
Finger
Heel
Ankle
Liver Yang
Sympathetic
Internal Tubercle
Knee
External Genital
Shenmen
Hip
Wrist
Sacral Vertebrae
Lumbo-sacral Vertebrae
Ischium
Buttock
Urethra
Urinary Bladder
Pancreas Kidney
Ureter
Gallbladder
Elbow
Appendix
Large Intestine
Liver
Chest
Duodenum
Thoracic Vertebrae
Lower Portion of Rectum
Small Intestine
Esophagus
Trachea
Cardiac Stomach
Spleen
Shoulder
Pharynx and Larynx
Heart
Nose
Lung
Cervical Vertebrae
Sanjiao
Brain
Clavicle
Internal Nose
Occiput
Forehead
Temple
Tongue
Face
Jaw
Cheek
Anterior Ear Lobe
Eye
Inner Ear
Tonsil

Back of Ear

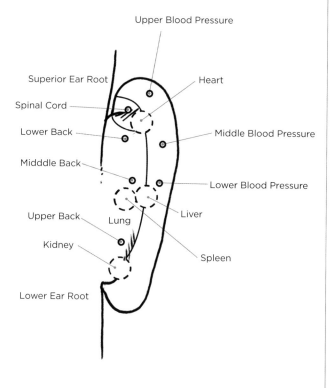

Upper Blood Pressure

Superior Ear Root

Heart

Spinal Cord

Lower Back

Middle Blood Pressure

Midddle Back

Lower Blood Pressure

Upper Back

Lung

Liver

Kidney

Spleen

Lower Ear Root

CONCLUSION

I applaud you for stepping forward to take control of your own healing. Each one of our paths is unique. My personal path led me through illness, accidents, and life-transforming events to greater health and balance, to becoming a healer and a teacher of healing practices. Your path may lead you to places you cannot even imagine right now.

As you embark on your own healing journey, I thank you for allowing me to help you walk down the path of Integrated Chinese Medicine. I fervently hope this book will inspire you to experience a life filled with wholeness and wellness as well as provide you with harmony of mind/body/spirit.

Your path may take you anywhere. There may be many turns or roadblocks. Sometimes the path may disintegrate before your eyes. Yet, when you go inside and pay close attention, you can visualize your internal path. That allows you to continue on the external one just a little bit farther, one step at a time.

About the Author

Misha Ruth Cohen, a doctor of Oriental medicine and licensed acupuncturist, is the clinical director of Chicken Soup Chinese Medicine, executive director of the Misha Ruth Cohen Education Foundation, and a former research specialist of Integrative Medicine at the University of California Institute for Health and Aging, all in San Francisco. She is a past member of the board of directors of the Society for Integrative Oncology and actively works in SIO committees. Dr. Cohen has been practicing traditional Asian medicine for the past forty-five years.

After attending Oberlin College, Misha Cohen was trained in acupuncture at Lincoln Hospital's Detox Program in the South Bronx under the auspices of the Quebec School of Acupuncture. Upon moving to California, she continued her studies in Chinese traditional medicine, acupuncture, and Chinese herbal medicine at the San Francisco College of Acupuncture and Oriental Medicine. She received her doctorate in gynecology from SFCAOM in 1987.

Dr. Cohen is nationally certified in acupuncture and herbal medicine by the National Certification Commission for Acupuncture and Oriental Medicine (NCCAOM). She has developed treatment protocols for people with HIV/AIDS, hepatitis C, liver disease, and cancer support. She was a member of the Ad Hoc Subpanel on Alternative and Complementary Therapy Research of the NIH Office of AIDS Research and in 1996 was selected by *POZ* magazine as one of fifty top AIDS researchers.

Dr. Cohen has written and been the subject of numerous professional and public oriented articles, has authored several peer-reviewed journal publications, has appeared on national radio and TV, and has published several books. She is the author of *The Chinese Way to Healing: Many Paths to Wholeness*, *The HIV Wellness Sourcebook: An East/West Guide to Living Well with HIV/AIDS and Related Conditions*, *The Hepatitis C Help Book*, and *The New Chinese Medicine Handbook*. She was the Complementary and Alternative Medicine Editor for *NUMEDX* magazine and was featured as a columnist in *Hepatitis Magazine/Liver Health Today* for several years.

Recognized internationally as a senior teacher and leading expert in Chinese traditional medicine, Dr. Cohen was invited several times by the Chinese government to present her programs, and her articles on HIV/AIDS were officially translated for use in China. Dr. Cohen currently is a faculty member at the American College of Traditional Chinese Medicine and teaches in various doctoral programs throughout the United States.

Dr. Cohen designed the HIV Professional Certification Program for Licensed Acupuncturists and the Hepatitis C Professional Training Program for Licensed Acupuncturists. She regularly trains Chinese medicine practitioners, including medical doctors, in Europe and the U.S.

She has presented her research projects at many scientific conferences, most notably the International AIDS Conference, the Society for Integrative Oncology, and the Society for Acupuncture Research.

Dr. Cohen has created Chinese medicine treatment protocols for PMS, infertility, hepatitis, HIV, endometriosis, HPV-related diseases, and menopausal syndromes that are used by many practitioners of Asian medicine. She has also developed herbal formulas for HIV, hepatitis C, chronic viral illness, cancer support, fibromyalgia, and the common cold.

Index